Current Clinical Pathology

Series Editor

Antonio Giordano
Philadelphia, PA, USA

This series includes monographs dealing with important topics in surgical pathology, cytopathology hematology, and diagnostic laboratory medicine. It is aimed at practicing hospital based pathologists and their residents providing them with concise up-to- date reviews and state of the art summaries of current problems that these physicians may encounter in their daily practice of clinical pathology.

More information about this series at http://www.springer.com/series/7632

Raf Sciot • Clara Gerosa • Gavino Faa
Editors

Adipocytic, Vascular and Skeletal Muscle Tumors

A Practical Diagnostic Approach

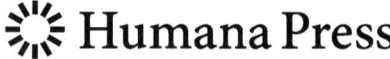 Humana Press

Editors
Raf Sciot
Department of Pathology
KU Leuven, UZ Gasthuisberg
Leuven, Belgium

Gavino Faa
Divisione di Anatomia Patologica
Dipartimento di Scienze Mediche e Sanità
Pubblica, Università degli Studi di Cagliari
Azienda Ospedaliero-Universitaria
di Cagliari
Cagliari, Italy

Clara Gerosa
Divisione di Anatomia Patologica
Dipartimento di Scienze Mediche e Sanità
Pubblica, Università degli Studi di Cagliari
Azienda Ospedaliero-Universitaria
di Cagliari
Cagliari, Italy

ISSN 2197-781X   ISSN 2197-7828   (electronic)
Current Clinical Pathology
ISBN 978-3-030-37459-4   ISBN 978-3-030-37460-0   (eBook)
https://doi.org/10.1007/978-3-030-37460-0

This Humana imprint is published by the registered company Springer Nature Switzerland AG
The registered company address is: Gewerbestrasse 11, 6330 Cham, Switzerland

Foreword

At the present time, seemingly in most countries throughout the world, the amount of teaching of both normal histology and pathology is significantly diminishing in medical school curricula. This means that when medical school graduates decide to pursue a career in pathology and begin their training, they have a very steep learning curve because much of what they see is entirely new to them and distinguishing between normal and pathological histology may also be a challenge. This is understandably stressful for all concerned and also means that pathologists-in-training have an enormous amount of information to learn during their usually 4- or 5-year training program.

Against this background, Professors Raf Sciot and Gavino Faa, with their colleagues, have devised a novel approach with the goal of facilitating pathology education or learning, in this volume specifically focused on three subsets of soft tissue tumors—those showing adipocytic, vascular or skeletal muscle differentiation. In addition to concise informative text and practical advice, the authors have included high-quality drawings of the salient histologic features of these various tumors, alongside photomicrographs, helping the relatively untrained or inexperienced eye to recognize the various structures or cell types that comprise each of these lesions. This innovative approach, which seeks to make recognition of these tumors easier, is clearly successful in its aim, as anyone reading through these pages will see. It is to be hoped (and anticipated!) that several additional volumes will follow, covering other areas of mesenchymal neoplasia—and it would not be difficult to imagine that other colleagues may seek to adopt a similar approach for other organ systems.

I believe that this first volume will be of considerable assistance to trainee pathologists and may well also be valuable for those already practicing pathology who have had limited exposure to soft tissue tumors. Professors Sciot and Faa and their colleagues are to be congratulated for introducing what may seem a very traditional, but practical, informative, and easy-to-use approach to pathology education.

Christopher D. M. Fletcher, M.D., FRCPath
Anatomic Pathology Brigham and Women's Hospital
Boston, MA, USA

Dana-Farber Cancer Institute
Boston, MA, USA

Harvard Medical School
Boston, MA, USA

Contents

Contributors

Maria Debiec-Rychter Department of Human Genetics, KU Leuven, UZ Gasthuisberg, Leuven, Belgium

Gavino Faa Divisione di Anatomia Patologica, Dipartimento di Scienze Mediche e Sanità Pubblica, Università degli Studi di Cagliari, Azienda Ospedaliero-Universitaria di Cagliari, Cagliari, Italy

Daniela Fanni Divisione di Anatomia Patologica, Dipartimento di Scienze Mediche e Sanità Pubblica, Università degli Studi di Cagliari, Azienda Ospedaliero-Universitaria di Cagliari, Cagliari, Italy

Giuseppe Floris Department of Pathology, KU Leuven, UZ Gasthuisberg, Leuven, Belgium

Clara Gerosa Divisione di Anatomia Patologica, Dipartimento di Scienze Mediche e Sanità Pubblica, Università degli Studi di Cagliari, Azienda Ospedaliero-Universitaria di Cagliari, Cagliari, Italy

Carlo Della Rocca Dipartimento di Scienze e Biotecnologie Medico-Chirurgiche, Policlinico Umberto I, Rome, Italy

Raf Sciot Department of Pathology, KU Leuven, UZ Gasthuisberg, Leuven, Belgium

Introduction

Regarding the interpretation of biopsies performed on soft tissue tumors, an old sentence of the philosopher Henry David Thoureau (1817–1862), "The question is not what you look at, but what you see," maintains during the years its value and fits perfectly with the difficulties encountered by pathologists in their daily clinical practice, in the diagnosis of these tumors. When sitting alone at the microscope looking at the hematoxylin and eosin (H&E)-stained sections of a soft tissue tumor, in such moments, it is not the complex chromosomal translocations we see, or the molecular changes underlying tumor insurgence and progression. It is the morphology of cells and their architecture, it are the characteristics of the stroma and of the vessels of the tumor, it is the tale of human pathology, the tradition of H&E that, probably, will never change. This will be the most complicated task of this book: in times in which molecular genetic approaches are an extremely relevant tool for the classification and therapy of soft tissue tumors, our aim is to underline the most important morphological and immunohistochemical data that should guide all surgical pathologists in the differential diagnosis of this family of tumors. To this end, in this book, we decided to focus on the use of drawings, utilized as vehicles for communicating the experiences of expert pathologists of previous generations to current surgical pathologists. Our idea is that a schematic representation of each tumor entity, and of all its variants, will help pathologists in training to build up their diagnostic skills, eventually reaching a correct diagnosis. Our goal is to provide better and faster training in the field of soft tissue tumors for resident pathologists, whose skill can mean the difference between life and death for patients. In addition, the most important molecular testing appropriate for each tumor entity will be reported, in an attempt to demonstrate the practical application of molecular analysis in the daily practice of surgical pathologists dealing with soft tissue tumors.

Adipocytic Tumors

1

Raf Sciot, Clara Gerosa, Daniela Fanni,
Maria Debiec-Rychter, and Gavino Faa

Introduction

Adipocytic tumors represent a heterogeneous group of soft tissue tumors, some of which are easily identified, thanks to the ability of tumor cells to differentiate along the lipomatous line, whereas others dedifferentiate to non-lipogenic neoplasms. Histology based on H&E-stained sections still represents the most essential tool for the diagnosis of the vast majority of adipocytic tumors, but in tumors that present diagnostic challenges at histology, cytogenetics and molecular genetics may play an important role in their diagnosis. Accurate gross sampling, proper orientation of the tumor, and identification of the closest margins – if possible – are the bases for a good diagnosis and estimation of prognosis.

From a practical point of view, the following suggestions might be useful:

1. Do not exclude an adipocytic origin when facing a spindle cell tumor without fat cells, particularly in a needle biopsy. If deep seated, it might be a dedifferentiated liposarcoma. Immunohistochemistry (MDM2) and FISH or CISH for amplification of *MDM2* should reveal the correct diagnosis. If superficial, it might be a spindle cell lipoma.
2. Do not automatically associate lipoblasts with the diagnosis of liposarcoma (LPS): lipoblasts may be absent in LPS, and they may be detected in benign lipomatous tumors, as well as in reactive conditions.

R. Sciot
Department of Pathology, KU Leuven, UZ Gasthuisberg, Leuven, Belgium

C. Gerosa · D. Fanni (✉) · G. Faa
Divisione di Anatomia Patologica, Dipartimento di Scienze Mediche e Sanità Pubblica, Università degli Studi di Cagliari, Azienda Ospedaliero-Universitaria di Cagliari, Cagliari, Italy

M. Debiec-Rychter
Department of Human Genetics, KU Leuven, UZ Gasthuisberg, Leuven, Belgium

© Springer Nature Switzerland AG 2020   1
R. Sciot et al. (eds.), *Adipocytic, Vascular and Skeletal Muscle Tumors*, Current Clinical Pathology, https://doi.org/10.1007/978-3-030-37460-0_1

3. When dealing with a mammary tumor, always consider silicon granuloma, often associated with leakeage of silicon from the fissured prosthesis and showing a high number of lipoblast-like macrophages.
4. In lipomatous tumors, infiltrative margins are not a sign of malignancy (see intramuscular lipoma).
5. The exact location of the tumor is often very informative. Facing a well-differentiated adipocytic tumor in the retroperitoneum, a well-differentiated LPS (lipoma-like) is most likely, and *MDM2* amplification should be searched for, by in situ hybridization-based techniques.
6. Nuclear pleomorphism in a fat tumor does not equal malignancy. Pleomorphic lipoma is a notable example.

Cell types occurring in lipomatous tumors (Fig. 1.1)

1. Mature adipocytes
2. Spindle cells
3. Lipoblasts
4. Floret-like multinucleated cells
5. Multivacuolated brown adipocytes
6. Bizarre hyperchromatic stromal cells
7. Pleomorphic lipoblasts

Lipoma (Fig. 1.2)

Definition It is the most frequent soft tissue tumor. It is generally solitary, but it may present as multiple tumors in +/− 5% of cases. It may be defined as a proliferation of mature adipocytes.

Age at Presentation Adults, 30–50 years.

Gender Men are more affected, particularly obese individuals.

Localization Lipomas may present in any anatomic location. When insurging in the retroperitoneum or in the abdomen, a well-differentiated liposarcoma (WDLPS) should always be considered first, given that benign lipomas in these locations are very rare. In other locations like the extremities and trunk, when a well-differentiated fatty lesion is deep-seated, more than 10 cm in diameter, and occurring in a patient older than 50 years, or the lesion is recurring, the possibility of an atypical lipomatous tumor (ALT) should always be considered and testing for MDM2 is mandatory (see chapter on ALT/WDLPS).

Clinical Presentation Painless, slow-growing mass of long duration. In deep lesions, the clinical presentation depends on the localization.

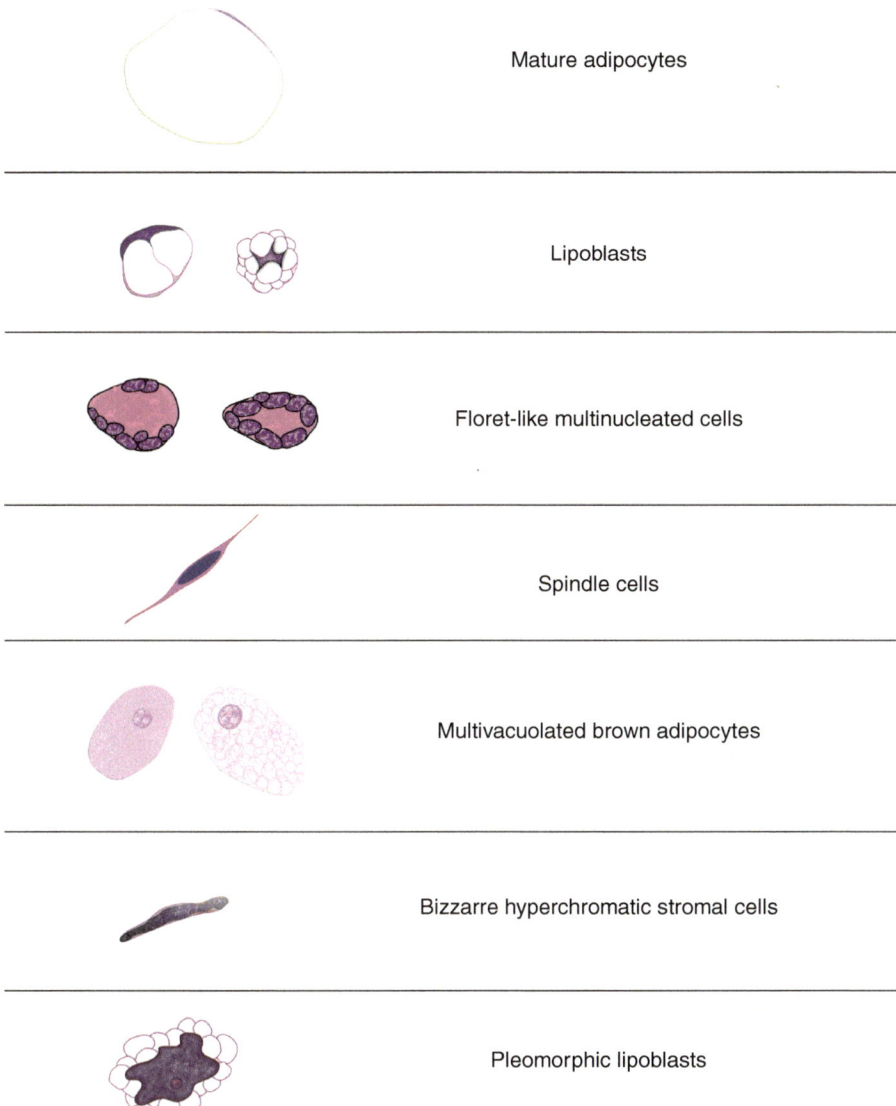

Mature adipocytes

Lipoblasts

Floret-like multinucleated cells

Spindle cells

Multivacuolated brown adipocytes

Bizzarre hyperchromatic stromal cells

Pleomorphic lipoblasts

Fig. 1.1 Cell types occurring in lipomatous tumors

Macroscopy Well-circumscribed mass – unless intramuscular – surrounded by a thin capsule, yellow on cut surface. Diameter ranges from 1 to 5 cm in superficial tumors, whereas deep tumors may reach larger dimensions.

Microscopy Proliferation of mature adipocytes. The size and shape of adipocytes are uniform, with minimal or no variation. Nuclei are small, inconspicuous, compressed at the cell periphery. Atypical nuclei or lipoblasts are generally absent.

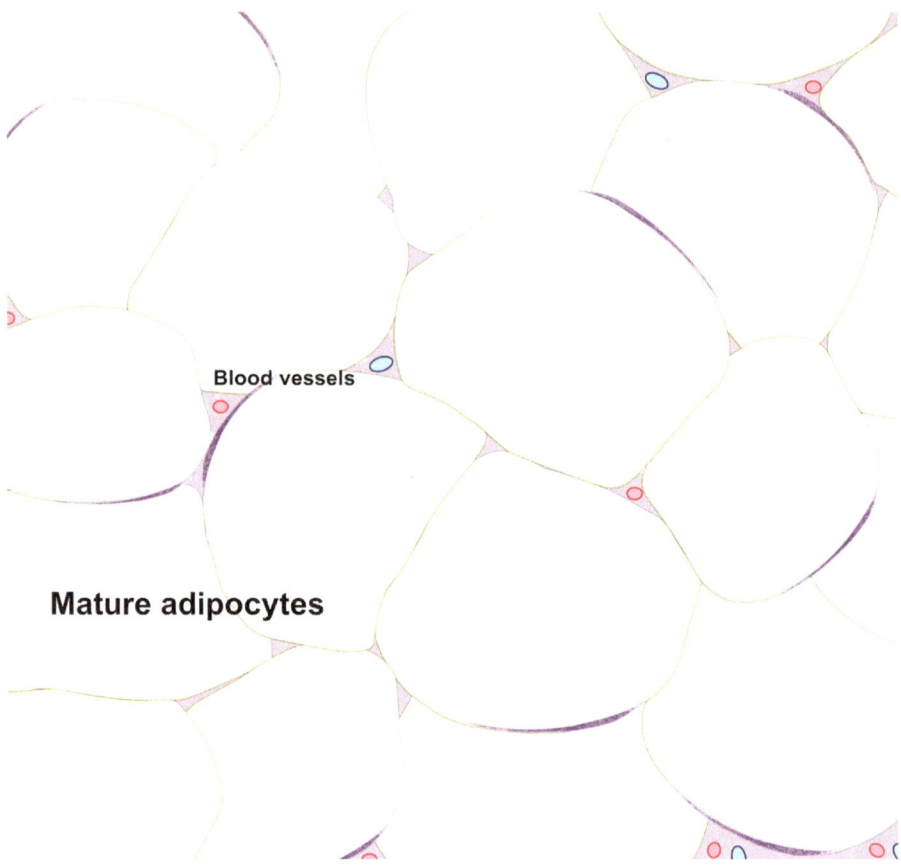

Fig. 1.2 Schematic representation of lipoma

Prominent nuclei with some atypia, associated with marked variation in size and shape of adipocytes, should lead to the suspicion of ALT/WDLPS. Focal fibrosis, fat necrosis, foamy histiocytes, multinucleated giant cells, and myxoid areas may be present.

Variants
(a) *Fibrolipoma.* Presence of foci of fibrosis and/or fibrous septa with spindle stromal cells. Adipocytes are characterized by uniformity in size and shape. Stromal cells do not show any atypia.
(b) *Myolipoma* (Fig. 1.3). Presence of bundles of mature desmin-positive smooth muscle cells (Fig. 1.4). It typically occurs in women in deep-seated locations (pelvis, retroperitoneum).
(c) *Myxoid lipoma.* Foci of myxoid stroma, scattered among adipocytes.
(d) *Intramuscular lipoma* (Fig. 1.5). Presence of atrophic striated fibers separated and infiltrated by adipocytes. It is characterized by a high rate of local recurrence, around 20%, when the involved muscle is not completely removed.

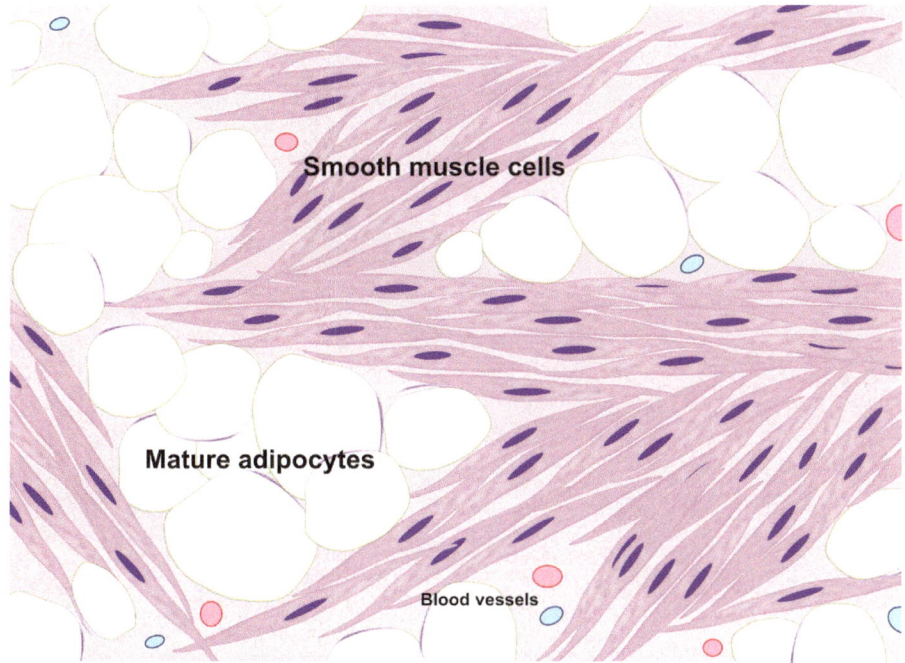

Fig. 1.3 Schematic representation of myolipoma

(e) *Lipomatosis.* A diffuse overgrowth of mature adipocytes, mainly localized in the subcutaneous regions, but occasionally extending to visceral organs. Some cases belong to the *PIKC3A* overgrowth syndromes.
   1. *Symmetric lipomatosis* (Madelung's disease). A massive lipomatous overgrowth localized in the neck region, which frequently infiltrates the underlying muscles.
   2. *Asymmetric lipomatosis.* A massive lipomatous overgrowth mainly localized in the extremities and trunk.
   3. *Pelvic lipomatosis.* Massive lipomatous overgrowth occupying the pelvis, leading to compression of the pelvic organs.
(f) *Osteolipoma* (Fig. 1.6). Presence of foci of metaplastic mature bone.
(g) *Chondrolipoma.* Presence of foci of metaplastic mature cartilage.

Immunohistochemistry Adipocytes in lipoma are S100-positive; however, in clinical practice, this stain does not play any role.

MDM2 and CDK4 expression in the nuclei of adipocytes and/or in spindle cells in the stroma exclude the diagnosis of lipoma.

Molecular Genetics 50% of adipocytic tumors carry an abnormal karyotype, including rearrangement of 12q13–15 or 6p21–23, or a deletion of 13q.

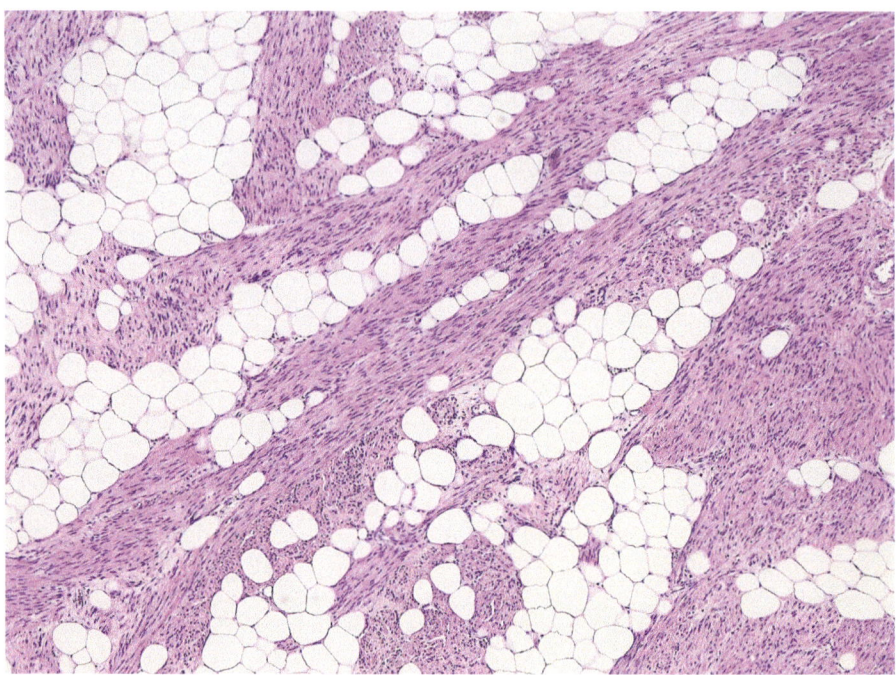

Fig. 1.4 Intraperitoneal myolipoma from a 51-year-old female (HE-stained section)

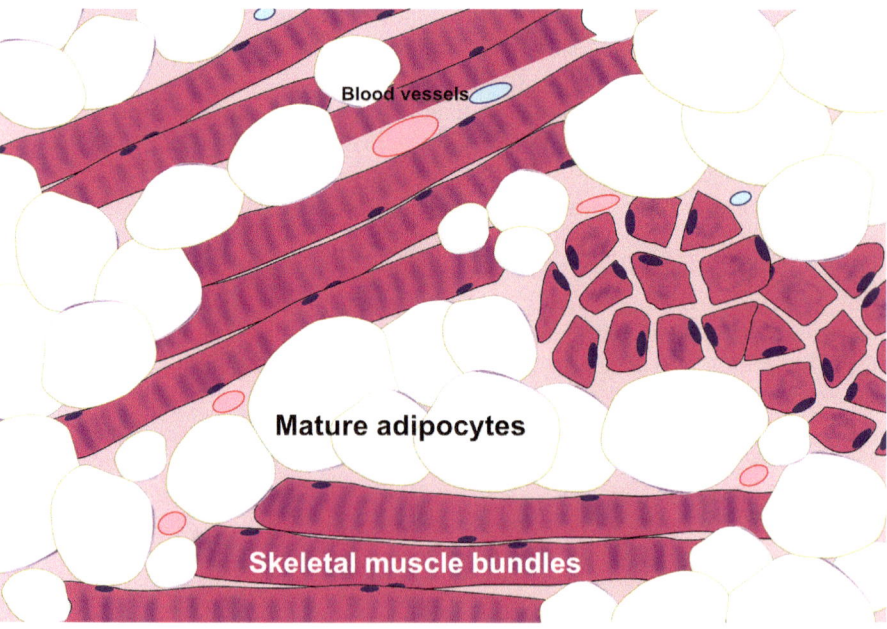

Fig. 1.5 Intramuscular lipoma (HE-stained section)

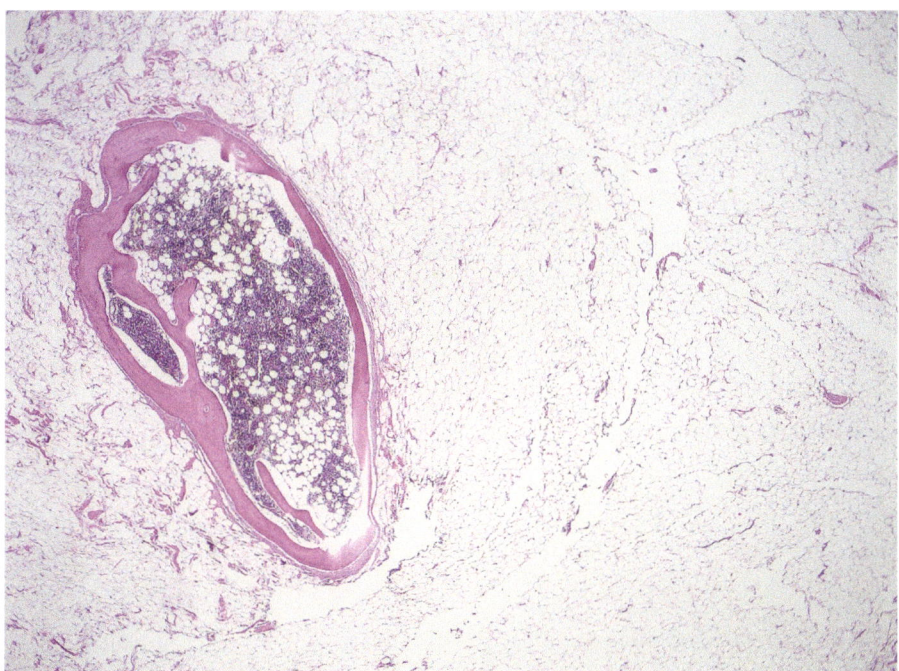

Fig. 1.6 Intermuscular osteolipoma from the arm of a 26-year-old female (HE–stained section)

Prognosis The complete excision of lipomas is curative.

Differential Diagnosis
1. *ALT/WDLPS:* absence of atypia in adipocytes and in stromal cells associated with uniformity of fat cells is in favor of lipoma. Nevertheless, in some instances, *MDM2* FISH should be done (see above in the section "Localization").
2. *Intramuscular hemangioma:* many intramuscular hemangiomas show a prominent adipocytic component.
3. *Fat necrosis:* it is often associated with marked variation in size of adipocytes, mimicking ALT/WDLPS.

Lipomatosis of Nerve (Fig. 1.7)

Definition Fibrolipomatous proliferation arising from the epineurium of a nerve.

Age at Presentation 10–30 years. It may be congenital.

Gender M = F

Localization Median nerve > ulnar >radial >peroneal >cranial nerves.

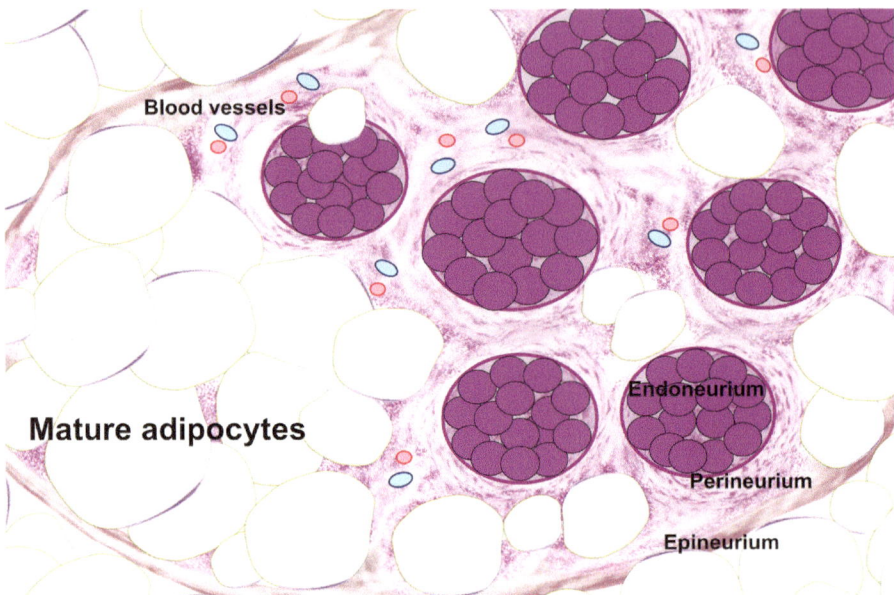

Fig. 1.7 Schematic representation of lipomatosis of nerve

Clinical Presentation (Fig. 1.8) Enlargement of the affected area, in about 50% associated with macrodactyly and/or compression neuropathy and local pain.

Macroscopy An epineurial firm mass, yellow on cut surface.

Microscopy (Fig. 1.9a, b) Mature adipocytes intermingled with a hypocellular fibrous component extending from the epineurium of the affected nerve. Perineural thickening can be seen as well.

Immunohistochemistry No significant diagnostic role.

Molecular Genetics No significant change. Rare *PIKC3A* mutations have been described.

Prognosis A wait-and-see approach and a nerve-sparing conservative approach are mandatory, given the functional damages which follow local excision.

Differential Diagnosis 1. Perineurioma: This differential diagnosis is restricted to rare cases of lipomatosis of nerve showing the pseudo-onion bulb pattern.

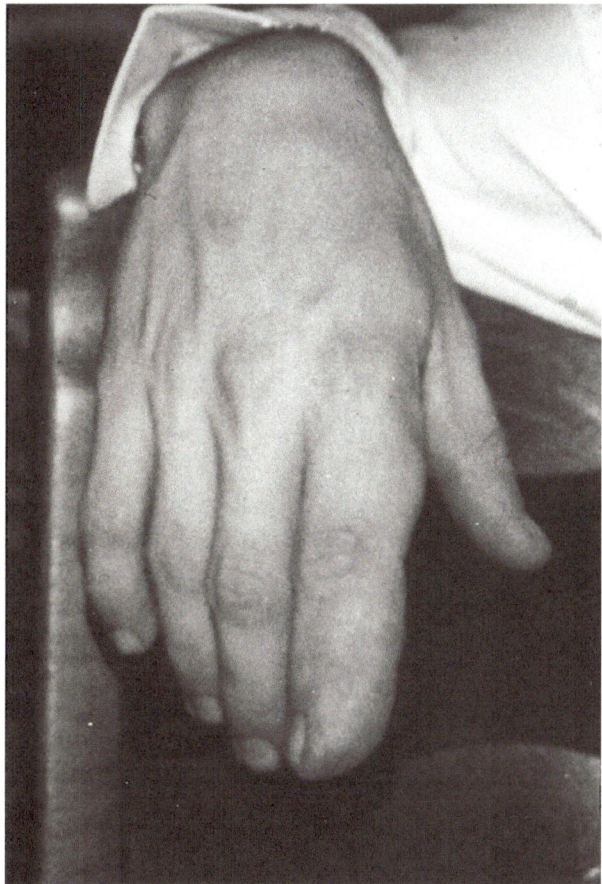

Fig. 1.8 Clinical picture of lipomatosis of nerve, showing the macrodactyly of the second finger

Angiolipoma (Fig. 1.10)

Definition Superficial tumor consisting of mature adipocytes and a capillary proliferation, with characteristic microthrombi.

Age at Presentation Young adults (20–30 years).

Gender Males predominate.

Localization Upper limbs (forearm) > trunk < lower limbs.

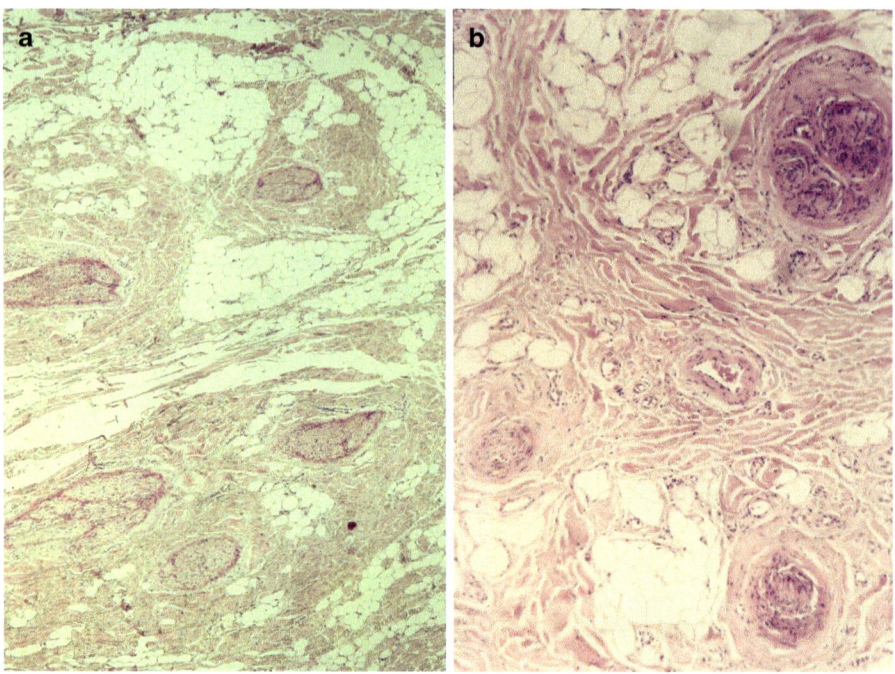

Fig. 1.9 Lipomatosis of nerve (**a, b**: HE-stained section), illustraing the fibro-fatty overgrowth in te epineurium

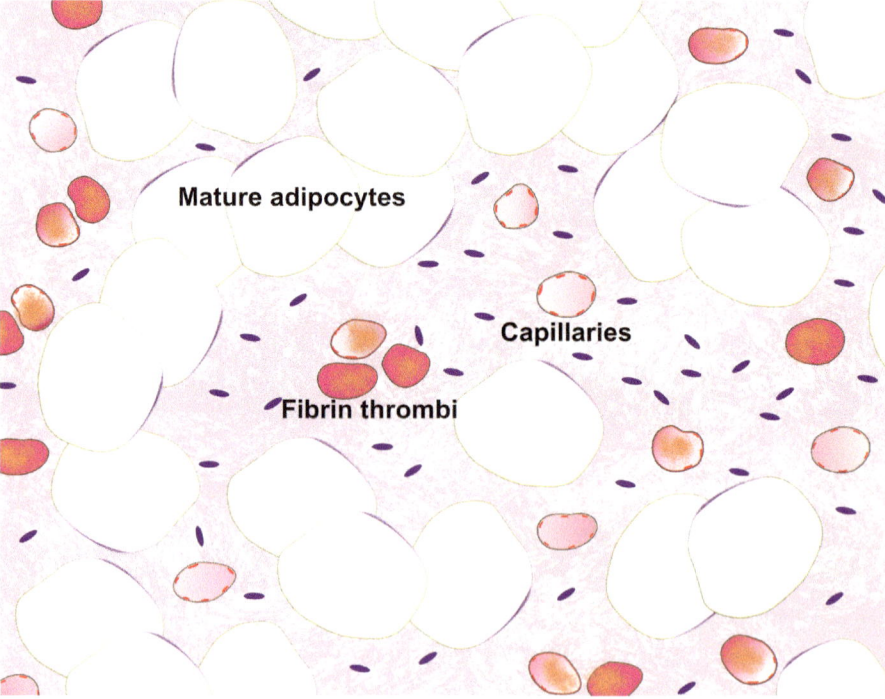

Fig. 1.10 Schematic representation of angiolipoma

Clinical Presentation Multiple (70%) subcutaneous (superficial) nodules, often painful.

Macroscopy Nodular lesion(s), well circumscribed with a capsule. On cut surface, yellow and reddish areas.

Microscopy (Fig. 1.11) Proliferation of mature adipocytes associated with a vascular network, consisting of capillaries. Fibrin microthrombi are frequently found.

Variants Cellular angiolipoma (Fig. 1.12): characterized by the predominance of the capillary component over the adipocytic component, simulating a vascular lesion.

Immunohistochemistry Does not play a significant role in this diagnosis.

Molecular Genetics A low level of protein *kinase D2* mutations has been described.

Prognosis Local excision is curative.

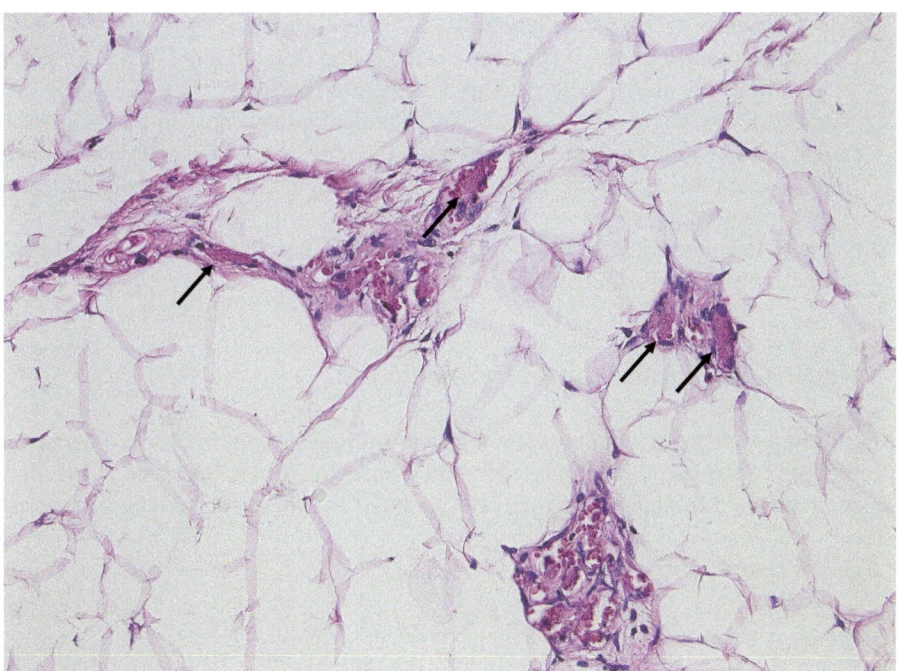

Fig. 1.11 Angiolipoma (HE-stained sections), arrows indicate microthrombi in capillary vessels

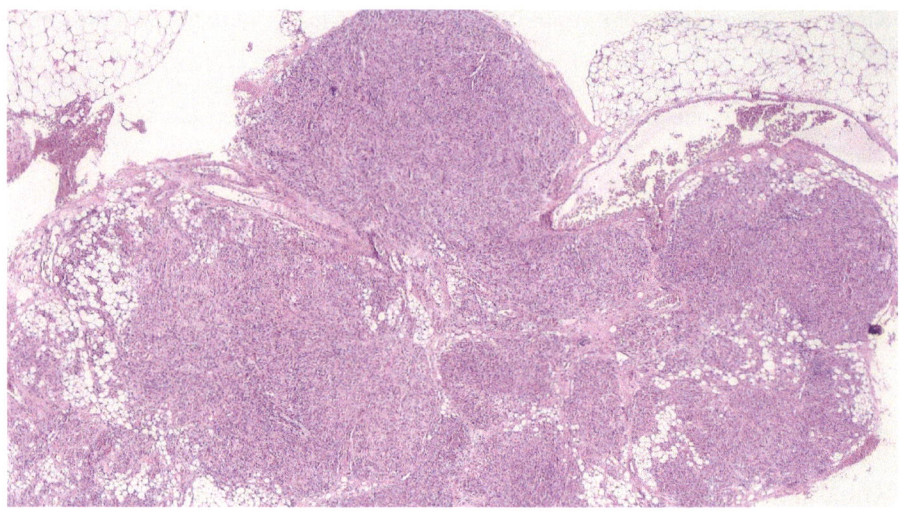

Fig. 1.12 Cellular angiolipoma from a 17-year-old male with multiple superficial lesions on the arm (HE stain)

Differential Diagnosis
1. Other *nodular lesions associated with pain* (angioleiomyoma, Schwannoma, glomus tumor, eccrine spiradenoma).
2. *Intramuscular angioma:* it is a deep-seated lesion (angiolipoma is always superficial), in which an adipocytic component is often present.
3. *Capillary hemangioma:* some capillary hemangiomas may show intervening adipocytes and may enter in the differential diagnosis with the cellular variant of angiolipoma. Microthrombi, typical of angiolipoma, are rare or absent in capillary hemangioma.
4. *Kaposi sarcoma:* may mimic a cellular angiolipoma, but shows more slit-like spaces and expresses human herpes virus 8 (HHV8).

Spindle Cell/Pleomorphic Lipoma (Fig. 1.13)

Definition Benign lipomatous tumor mainly occurring subcutaneously in older males, composed of a mixture of spindle cells and adipocytes, which may exhibit cytologic pleomorphism. Multinucleated giant cells are often present in the pleomorphic variant.

Age at Presentation >55 years.

Gender Male predominance (M/F = 10/1).

Localization Neck > upper back (shoulder) > face > oral cavity. Only rarely described outside the head and neck and back regions.
    Solitary > multiple.

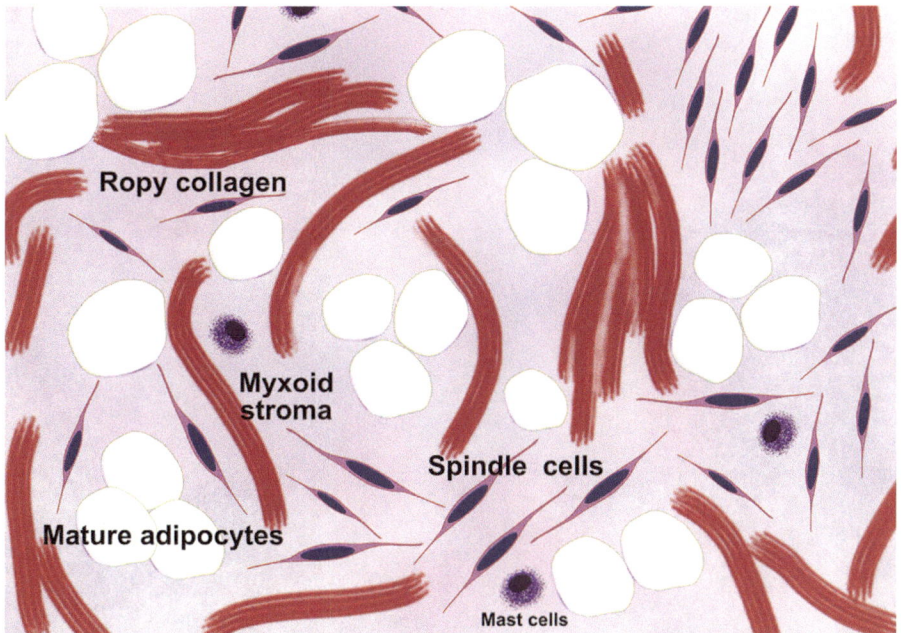

Fig. 1.13 Schematic representation of spindle cell lipoma

Clinical Presentation Superficial, mainly subcutaneous painless tumor.

Macroscopy Two components: one yellow, the other white-gray.

Microscopy (Fig. 1.14) A variable amount of bland spindle cells and mature adipocytes in a fibro-myxoid stroma is seen. Dense hyper-eosinophilic collagen bundles (ropy collagen fibers) are characteristic. There may be variation in adipocyte size and bizarre hyperchromatic cells. If numerous multinucleated giant cells with a floret-like appearance are present, the term pleomorphic lipoma is used. Occasional lipoblasts can be present. Some cases are poor in fat cells.

Variants
A. *Dermal.* Purely dermal, may occur outside the head and neck and back regions.
B. *Cellular.* Predominance of spindle cells, with rare intermingled adipocytes. Spindle cells show uniform nuclei. Isolated atypical cells, with enlarged hyperchromatic nuclei may be observed.
C. *Myxoid/angiomatoid.* Extensive myxoid stroma, angiectoid spaces (Fig. 1.15).
D. *Atypical spindle/pleomorphic lipoma* Presence of atypical spindle cells, variability in adipocyte size, pleomorphic lipoblasts, and poor circumscription. Lesions can recur but do not metastasize. This variant is considered to be a separate entity in the recent (2020) WHO classification.

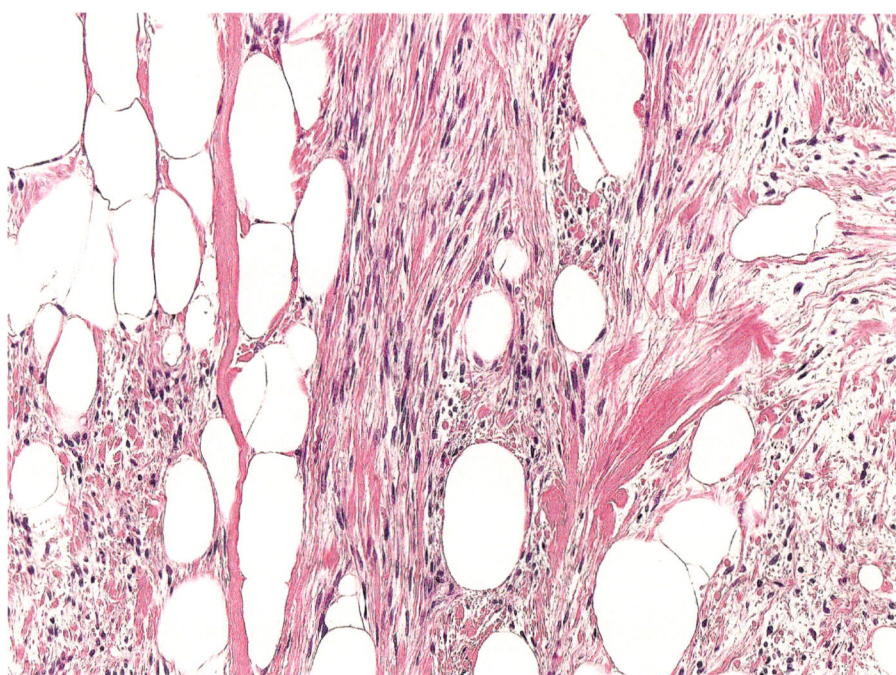

Fig. 1.14 Spindle cell lipoma (HE-stained sections), highlighting the spindle cells and ropy collagen

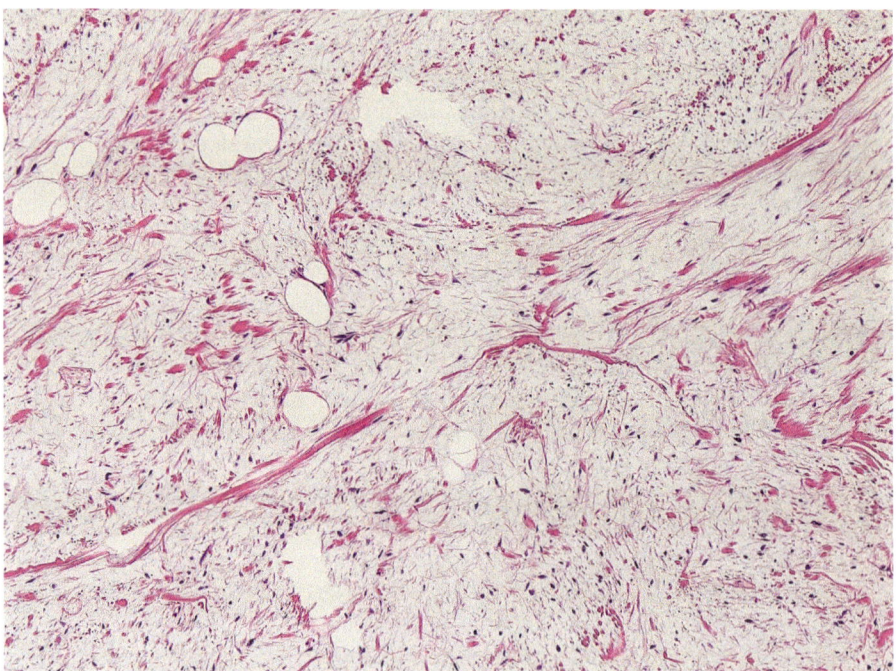

Fig. 1.15 Myxoid spindle cell lipoma (HE-stained sections)

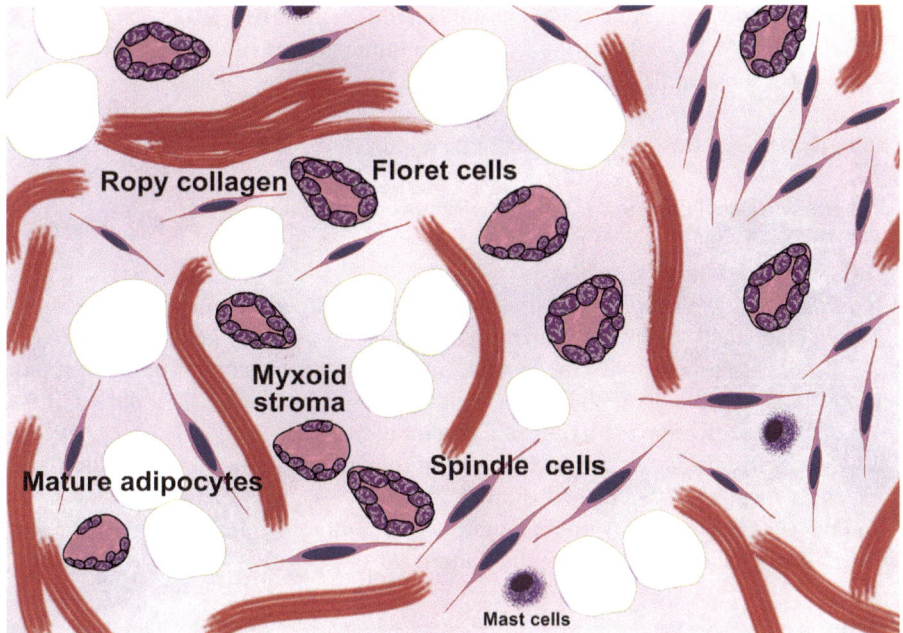

Fig. 1.16 Schematic representation of pleomorphic lipoma

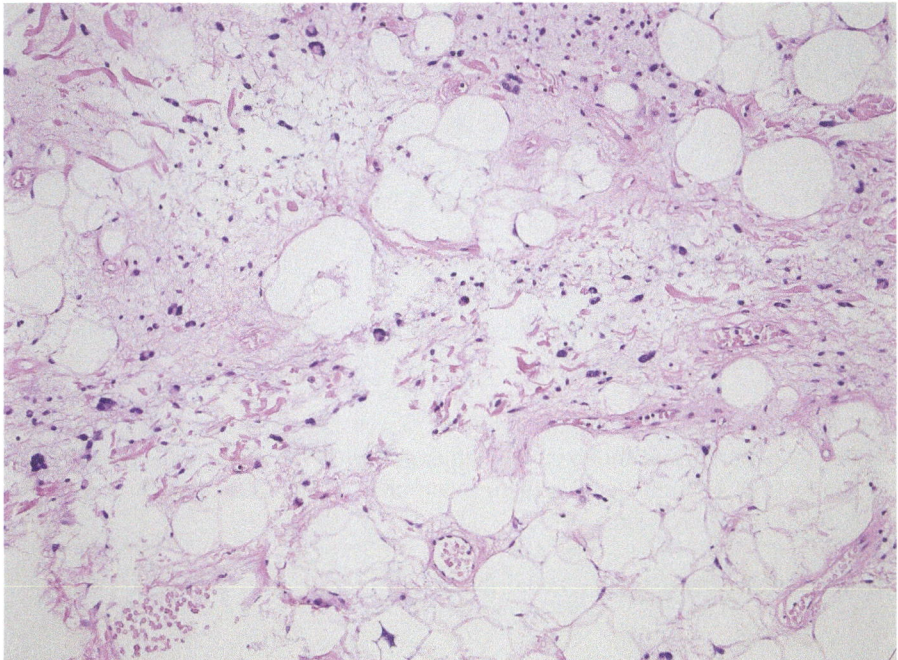

Fig. 1.17 Pleomorphic lipoma from the subcutaneous tumor of the neck in an 82-year-old male (HE-stained sections), showing the multinucleated giant cells and ropy collagen

Immunohistochemistry CD34+ (strong and diffuse), CD10+, S100−, alpha-smooth muscle actin (SMA)−, desmin −. Loss of Rb immunoreactivity indicates 13q14 loss. Adipocytes and spindle cells are always MDM2−.

Molecular Genetics 13q14 or 16q22 deletion.

Prognosis Local excision is curative. Recurrences extremely rare.

Differential Diagnosis
1. *Mammary-type myofibroblastoma:* tumor occurring along the milkline containing bland and more fascicular myofibroblast-type cells and less adipocytes. There is strong reactivity for desmin. Since myofibroblastoma, spindle cell/pleomorphic lipoma, and cellular angiofibroma have the same 13q14 deletion, they can be considered phenotypes of a common disease.
2. *Myxoid liposarcoma*: deep-seated tumor, plexiform "crow's feet" capillary network; specific *FUS/DDIT3* fusion.
3. *Low-Grade Myxofibrosarcoma*: multinodular, more atypical pleomorphic tumor cells, typical curvilinear vascular pattern.

Hemosiderotic Fibrolipomatous Tumor (HFLT) (Fig. 1.18)

Definition Benign tumor characterized by the proliferation of spindle cells and adipocytes in a hemosiderotic background, with a high rate of recurrence (30–50%).

Age Middle age (40–50 years).

Gender Mainly women.

Localization Ankle region > upper limbs > hands > head and neck.

Clinical Course Subcutaneous tumor.

Macroscopy Unencapsulated nodule, yellow on cut surface, with well-defined margins, 2–10 cm in diameter.

Microscopy (Fig. 1.19) Bland spindle fibroblast-like cells associated with mature adipocytes, fibroblasts, mononuclear inflammatory cells, and abundant hemosiderin granules both in tumor cells and in macrophages. Pleomorphism is focal, when present. Mitoses are scarce.

Immunohistochemistry Not contributive.

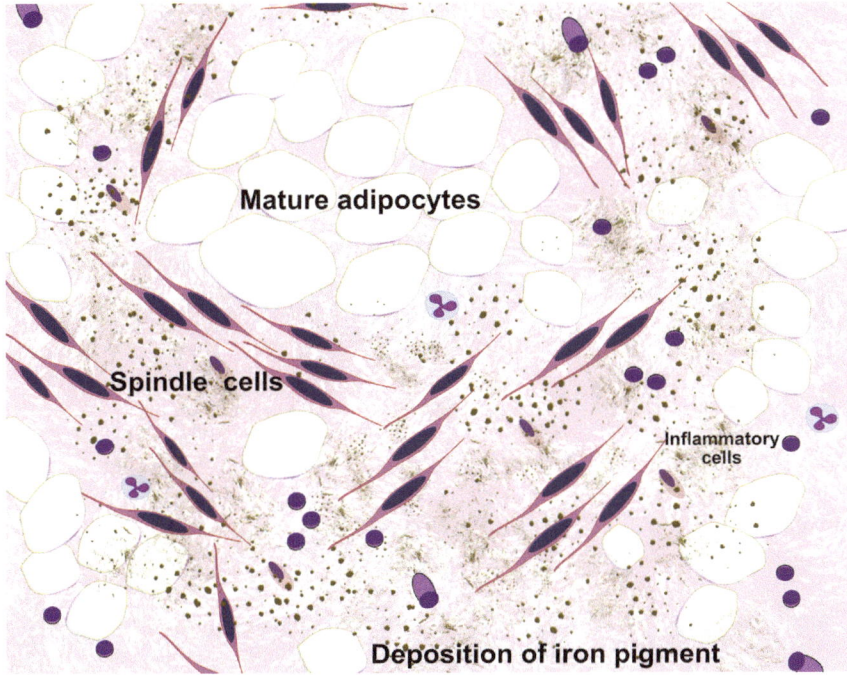

Fig. 1.18 Schematic representation of hemosiderotic fibrolipomatous tumor

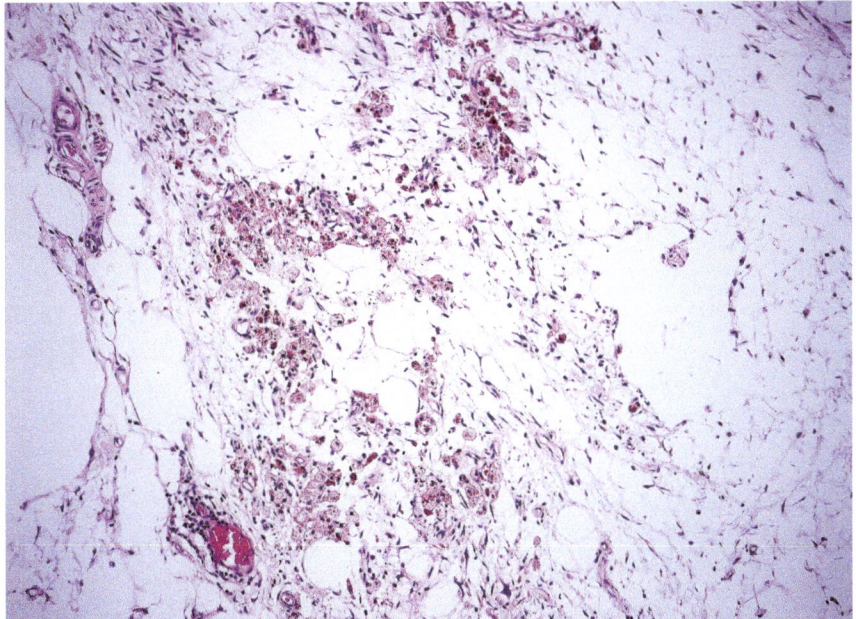

Fig. 1.19 Hemosiderotic fibrolipomatous tumor from a 48-year-old female with a subcutaneous tumor of the hip (HE-stained sections), composed of mature adipocytes, inflammatory cells and hemosiderin loaded macrophages

Molecular Genetics Reciprocal translocations involving chromosomes 1 and 10, causing rearrangements of the *TGFBR3* and *MGEA5* genes. The same change is seen in myxoinflammatory fibroblastic sarcoma.

Prognosis No metastatic potential, but high recurrence rate.

Lipoblastoma (Fig. 1.20)

Definition Benign adipocytic tumor of infancy and early childhood that recapitulates adipose tissue differentiation during fetal life.

Age <3 years of life in 75–90% of cases.

Gender Mainly males

Localization Trunk, extremities (lower and upper) > mediastinum >retroperitoneum.

Clinical Presentation Well-demarcated nodule or diffuse infiltrative mass (lipoblastomatosis), slowly growing, painless.

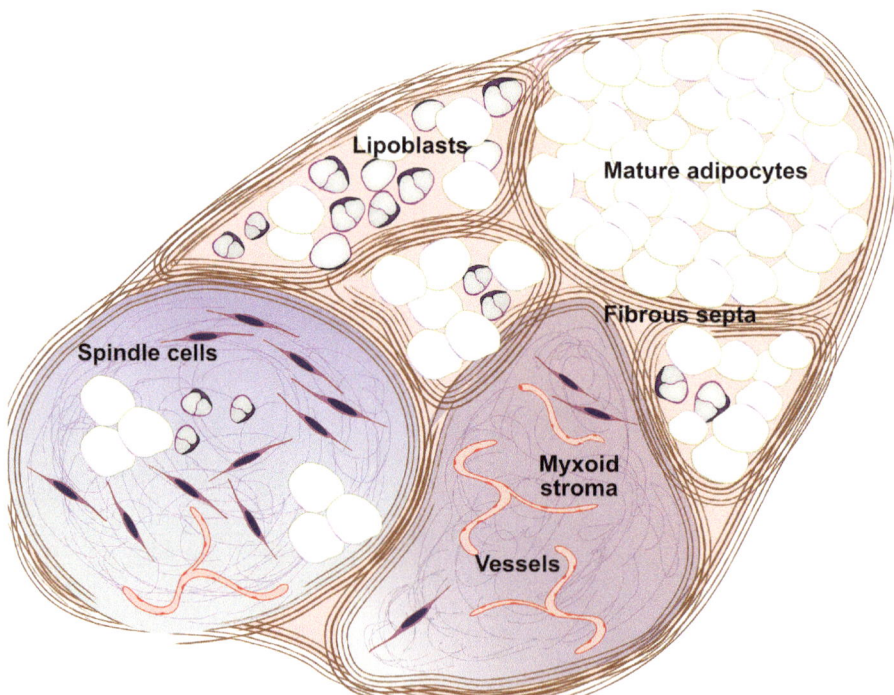

Fig. 1.20 Schematic representation of lipoblastoma

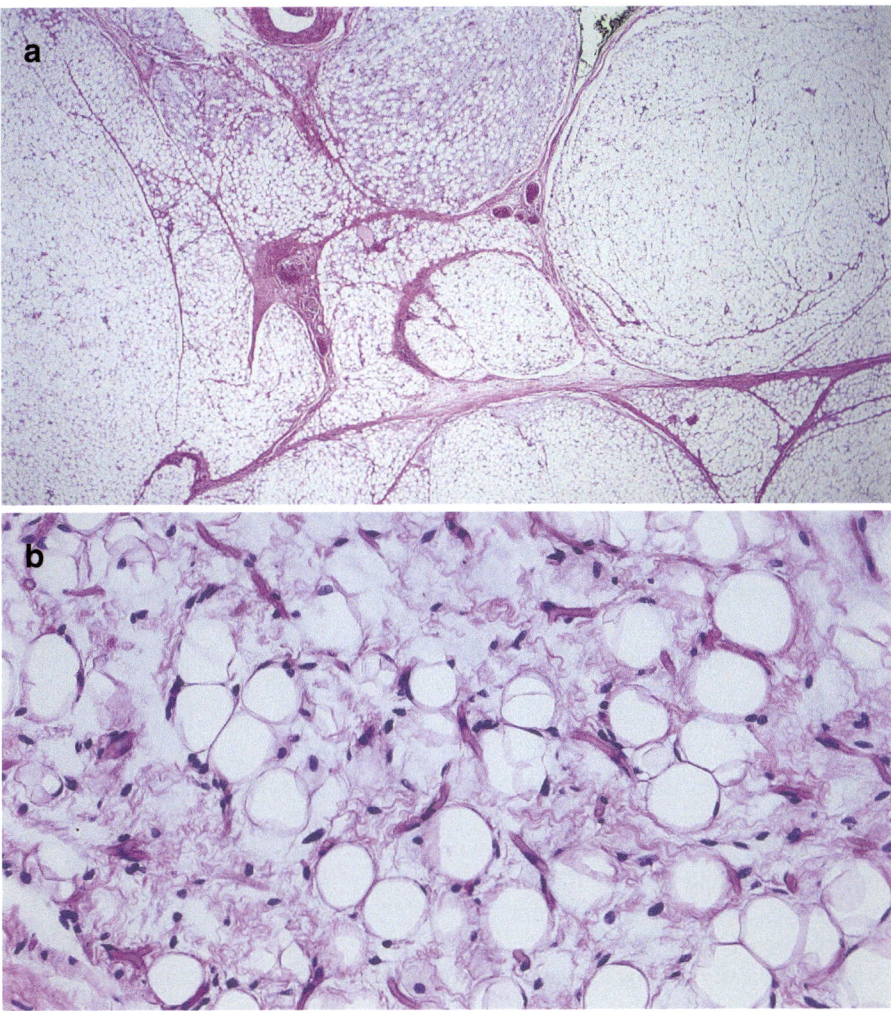

Fig. 1.21 Lipoblastoma from the neck of a 3-year-old boy at low-power (**a**) and high-power (**b**) field magnification (HE-stained sections), illustrating the lobulation, the myxoid matrix and branching vessels, mimicking myxoid liposarcoma

Macroscopy Lobulated cut surface, white-yellow.

Microscopy (Fig. 1.21a, b) Lobules of mature adipocytes, separated by thin fibrous septa, intermingled with lipoblasts and immature spindle cells (preadipocytes). Occasionally, the stroma can be very myxoid. Multivacuolated lipoblasts are often numerous. Thin vessels can give rise to a plexiform vascular pattern (as in myxoid liposarcoma).

Immunohistochemistry Not contributive.

Molecular Genetics Rearrangement of the 8q11–13 region; fusion genes: *HAS2/PLAG1* and/or *COL1A2/PLAG1*.

Differential Diagnosis
1. *Ordinary lipoma*: lacks the lipoblasts.
2. *Myxoid liposarcoma*: age > 10 years, no prominent lobular pattern, *FUS/DDIT3* fusion gene.

Prognosis Complete excision is curative, recurrences occur in 13–46% of patients (not restricted to diffuse lipoblastomatosis).

Angiomyolipoma (AML)

Definition It is a member of PEComas, a group of neoplasms with perivascular epithelioid cell differentiation, mainly occurring in women.

Age at Presentation Middle-aged patients (45–55 years) in sporadic cases; 25–35 when associated with tuberous sclerosis.

Gender Females predominate (F/M = 4/1).

Localization Kidney > retroperitoneum > liver > oral cavity > lungs.

Clinical Course Sporadic > associated with tuberous sclerosis.

Macroscopy Unencapsulated mass with infiltrative margins. On cut surface, hemorrhagic areas and necrotic foci may be present.

Microscopy (Fig. 1.22) Multiple cell components: (a) angio: thick-walled blood vessels, typically lacking an elastica. (b) myo: spindle to epithelioid smooth muscle-like cells; (c) lipo: mature adipocytes. Lipoblasts may be present.

Variants Monotypical epithelioid to spindled variants: solid islands of large polygonal epithelioid to spindled cells with eosinophilic or clear cytoplasm, organized in nests or sheets surrounded by a delicate capillary network. Mature adipocytes are only focal or absent. Broad fibrous septa, intermingled with the sheets of epithelioid cells, may be detected in some tumor areas ("sclerosing pecoma").

Immunohistochemistry Co-expression of melanocytic markers (HMB45, Melan-A, Microphtalmia transcription factor (MITF)) and smooth muscle markers (alpha-SMA, calponin) is typical.

Molecular Genetics Non-clonal chromosomal changes. *TSC-2* mutations or deletions. 15% of pecomas have *TFE3* rearrangement.

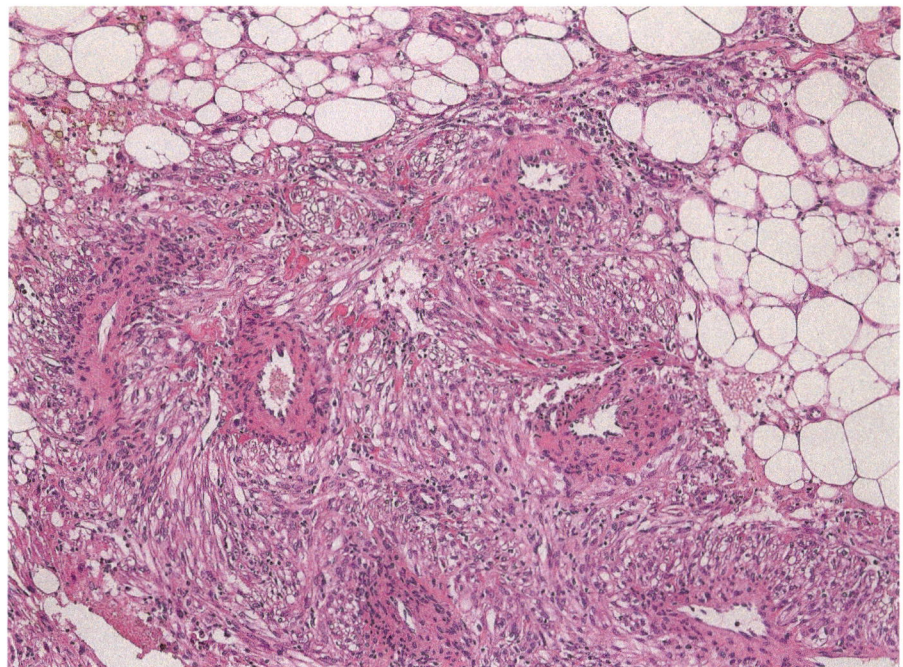

Fig. 1.22 Angiomyolipoma (HE-stained sections), illustrating the three components

Prognosis Conventional typical AML is virtually always benign. Epithelioid renal and extrarenal AML has metastatic potential (lungs, bone, liver) but the behavior is hard to predict.

Differential Diagnosis
1. *Renal cell carcinoma*: diffuse reactivity for keratin and EMA
2. *Epithelioid melanoma*: strong S100 immunostaining, no muscle markers
3. *Rhabdomyosarcoma*: expression of desmin and myogenin
4. *Epithelioid leiomyosarcoma*: diffuse reactivity for h-caldesmon, negativity for S100 and other melanocytic markers
5. *Epithelioid sarcoma*: loss of INI1 expression, reactivity for CD34 and keratin
6. *Gastrointestinal stromal tumor (GIST)*: DOG1+, CD117+
7. *Alveolar soft part sarcoma (ASPS):* no melanocytic markers

Myelolipoma (Fig. 1.23)

Definition Benign adipocytic tumor consisting of adipocytes admixed with hematopietic elements.

Age Mid to adult life.

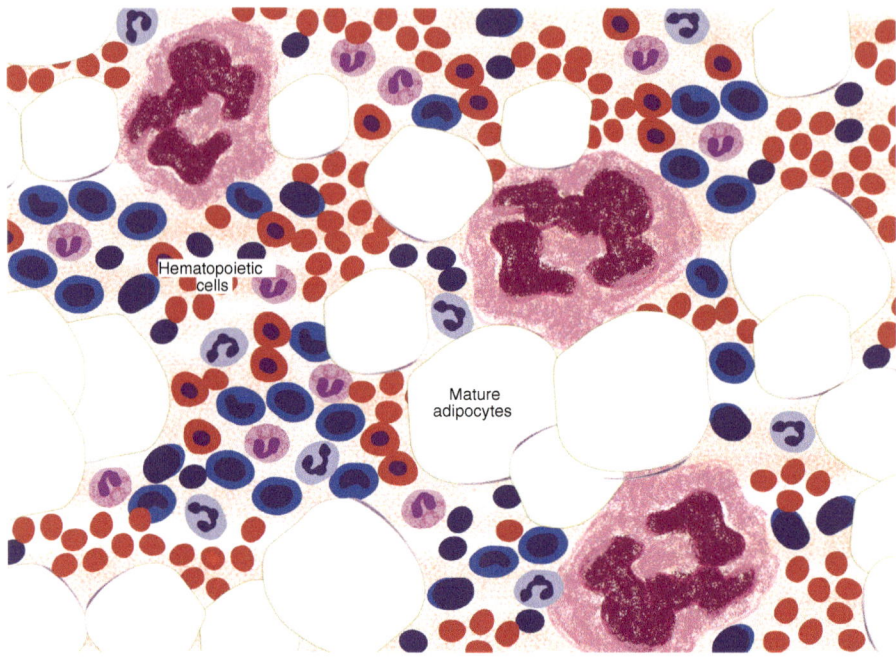

Fig. 1.23 Schematic representation of myelolipoma

Gender No sex predominance.

Localization The adrenal gland is by far the most frequent site.

Clinical Presentation Nodule in the adrenal gland. Often coincidental finding.

Macroscopy Well-circumscribed, lobulated cut surface, yellow–grayish red.

Microscopy (Fig. 1.24) Mature fat admixed with a variable amount of bone marrow elements.

Immunohistochemistry Not contributive.

Molecular Genetics A t(3;21)(q25;p11) has been described.

Prognosis Local excision is curative.

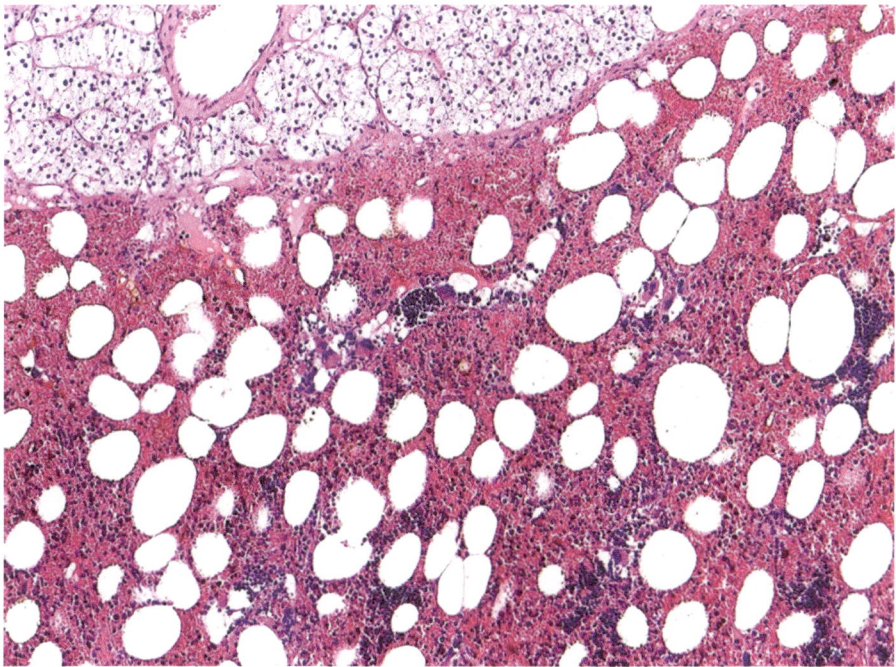

Fig. 1.24   Myelolipoma. The tumor consists of hemorrhagic hematopietic tissue and mature fat. A rim of adrenocortical tissue is still seen

Hibernoma (Fig. 1.25)

Definition   Benign adipocytic tumor with predominant brown multivacuolated adipocytes.

Age   Young adults (20–40 years).

Gender   Slight male predominance.

Localization   Thigh > trunk > upper limbs > head and neck.

Clinical Presentation   Superficial or deep-seated nodule.

Macroscopy   Well-circumscribed, lobulated cut surface, yellow to red-brown in color.

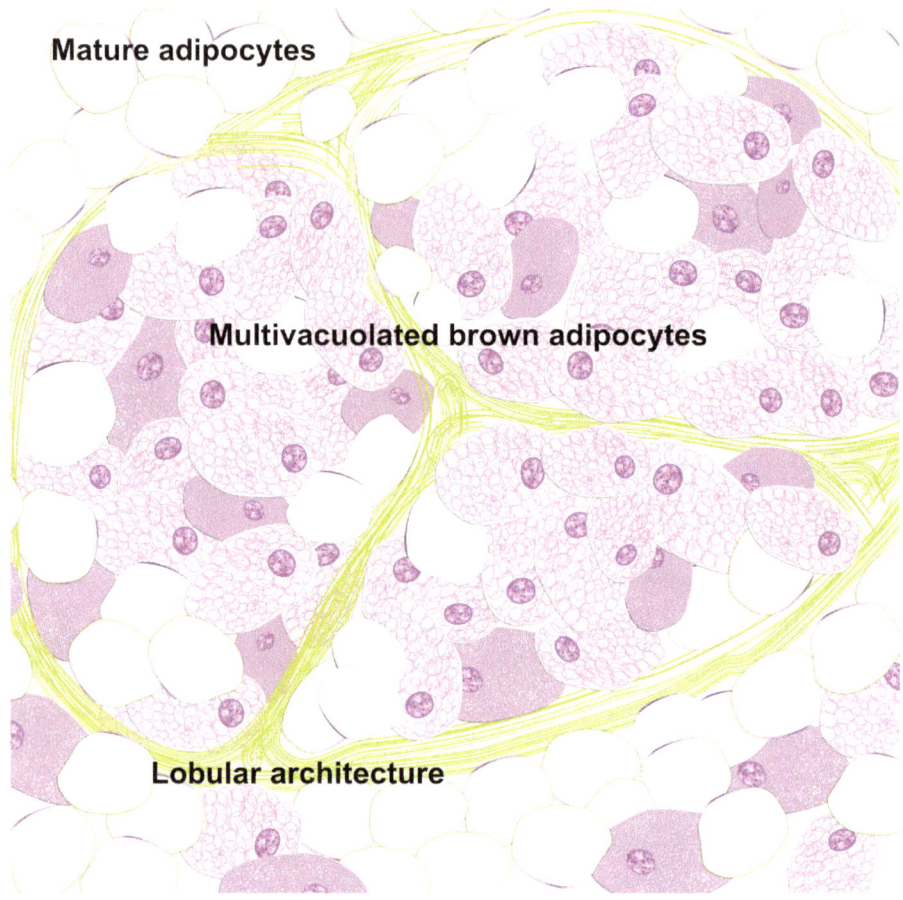

Fig. 1.25 Schematic representation of hibernoma

Microscopy (Fig. 1.26) Lobular architecture; multivacuolated adipocytes, with granular cytoplasm and central round nuclei; mature adipocytes; eosinophilic granular cells; focal myxoid stroma; no atypia, no mitoses.

Variants In rare cases, the histological picture is characterized by the prevalence of mature adipocytes, encircling a minority of scattered multivacuolated adipocytes with granular cytoplasm, isolated or in small groups.

Immunohistochemistry Not contributive

Molecular Genetics Rearrangement of the 11q13–21 region; deletion of the *MEN1/AIP* gene.

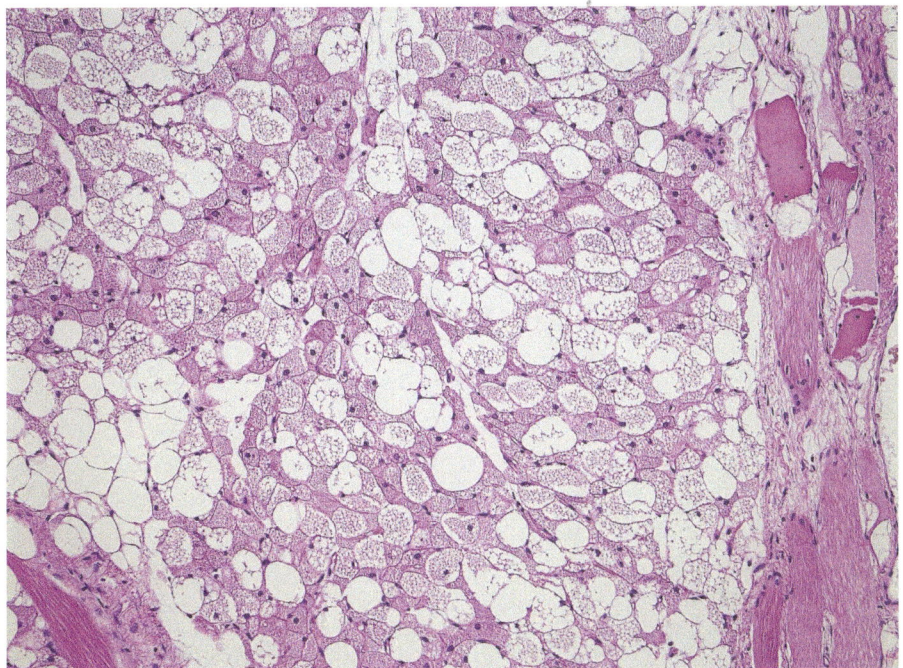

Fig. 1.26 Hibernoma from the deep-seated tumor of the upper leg in a 40-year-old female (HE-stained section)

Prognosis Local excision is curative.

Differential diagnosis *ALT/WDLPS*. Some hibernomas are characterized by a predominant component of large multivacuolated lipoblast-like cells. A negative staining for MDM2 and CDK4, associated with the absence of MDM2 amplification, allows for the correct diagnosis of hibernoma.

Chondroid Lipoma (Fig. 1.27)

Definition Very rare benign adipocytic tumor characterized by a mixture of mature adipocytes, chondroblast-like cells, eosinophilic granular cells and lipoblasts, in a myxochondroid background.

Age 20–30 years.

Gender More frequent in women.

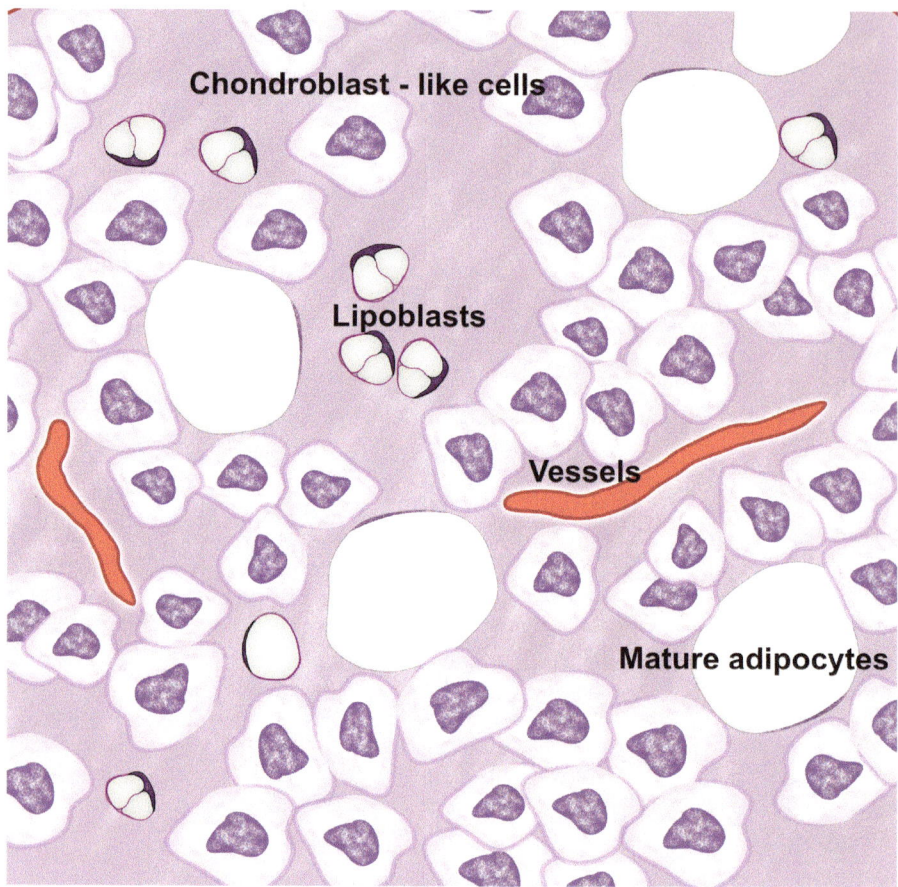

Fig. 1.27 Schematic representation of chondroid lipoma

Localization   Proximal limbs, limb girdles, trunk, extremities, head and neck.

Clinical Presentation   Deep, painless, slow-growing mass. 20% may be superficial.

Macroscopy   Encapsulated, multilobular in 30% of cases, white-yellow on cut surface.

Microscopy (Fig. 1.28a, b)   Mature adipocytes, chondroblast-like cells, lipoblasts, cells with eosinophilic granular cytoplasm, myxochondroid background, lobular pattern, thick-walled blood vessels.

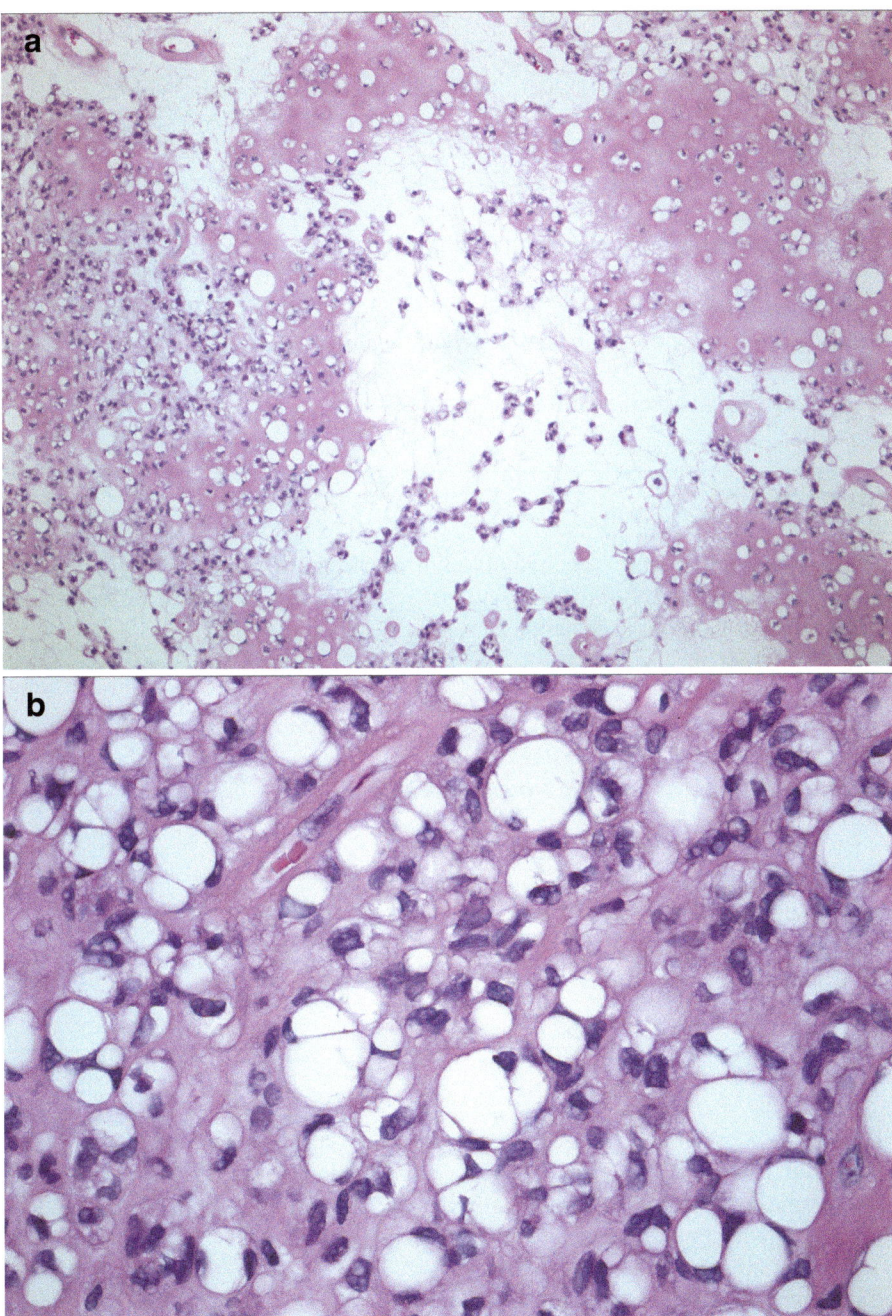

Fig. 1.28 Chondroid lipoma from a 71-year-old male with an incidentally found lesion in the spinal erector muscle at low-power (**a**) and high-power (**b**) field magnification (HE-stained sections), showing the myxochondroid background and the lipoblasts

Immunohistochemistry S100+.

Molecular Genetics t(11;16)(q13;p13). Fusion genes: *C11orf95-MRTFB*

Differential Diagnosis
1. *Soft tissue chondroma:* mainly localized in hands and feet; composed of true hyaline cartilage
2. *Myxoid liposarcoma:* plexiform capillary vascular pattern; myxoid but no chondroid appearance
3. *Soft tissue myoepithelioma:* immunostaining for keratin, EMA, GFAP, or S100
4. *Chondrolipoma:* presence of mature cartilage in a lipoma

Prognosis Surgical removal is curative

Liposarcoma

Definition Malignant mesenchymal tumor, showing diffuse or only partial adipocytic differentiation, ranging from low-grade lesions with only recurrence potential to metastasizing high-grade neoplasms, depending on the subtype.

Major Subtypes
1. *Atypical lipomatous tumor (ALT)/well-differentiated liposarcoma (WDLPS)*
2. *Dedifferentiated LPS (DDLPS)*
3. *Myxoid/high-grade myxoid (round cell) LPS*
4. *Pleomorphic LPS*

Major Cytogenetic Findings: Fig. 1.29a–c
1. Amplification of *MDM2/CDK4* (ALT/WDLPS; DDLPS)
2. Rearrangement of *FUS/DDIT3* (Myxoid LPS)
3. Complex karyotypic aberrations (pleomorphic LPS)

ALT/WDLPS

Definition Low-grade, locally aggressive well-differentiated malignant fatty tumor. ALT is often used to delineate lesions occurring in surgically amenable sites (extremities), WDLPS for biologically exactly the same tumor in the retroperitoneum or mediastinum (higher morbidity/mortality).

Frequency 40–45% of all LPS (the largest subgroup).

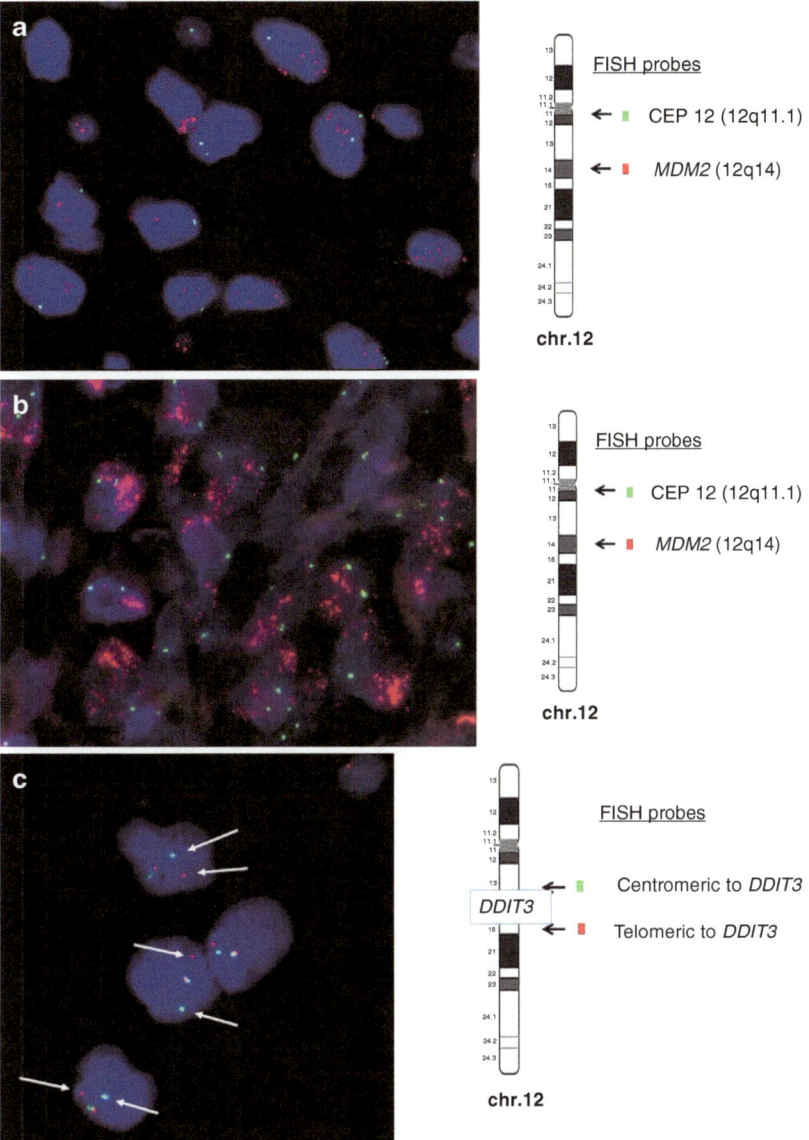

Fig. 1.29 (**a**) Example of FISH image of atypical lipoma immunonegative for MDM2, showing low-level amplification of *MDM2* (from 2 to 12 red signals per nuclei), as detected by the co-hybridization of SpectrumOrange labeled *MDM2* and SpectrumGreen labeled chromosome 12 centromeric (CEP) probes; (**b**) dual-color inter-phase FISH image in dedifferentiated liposarcoma, showing high-level amplification of *MDM2* (>90% of nuclei), as detected by the co-hybridization of SpectrumOrange labeled MDM2 (red signals) and SpectrumGreen labeled chromosome 12 centromeric CEP (green signals) probes; (**c**) interphase dual color FISH detection of *DDIT3* rearrangement as evidenced by overlapping, green/red signals (normal), associated with the split red and green signals from the probe that flank *DDIT3* gene (arrows) in tumor nuclei

Age at Presentation Adults >40 years.

Localization Limbs, retroperitoneum, paratesticular region (spermatic cord), mediastinum, head and neck.

Clinical Course Slow growing mass, often reaching a large size.

Macroscopy Yellow (lipomatous component), white-gray areas (fibrosis).

Microscopy Four main subtypes of ALT/WDLPS have been described:

A. *Lipoma-like subtype* (Fig. 1.30). Mature adipocytes are the principal constituent of this subtype. Fat cells show marked variation in size and at least focal nuclear atypia. Fibrous septa may be found, including spindle cells with hyperchromatic nuclei and focal atypical nuclei. Uni- or multivacuolated lipoblasts may be detected, but they are not a constant finding and are not required for the diagnosis (Fig. 1.31).
B. *Sclerosing subtype* (Fig. 1.32). The constant finding is represented by a fibrillary collagenous background, with bizarre hyperchromatic stromal cells. Adipocytes are patchy, so the lipogenic features may be overlooked in needle biopsies. Lipoblasts may be detected, mainly the multivacuolated ones (Fig. 1.33).
C. *Inflammatory subtype* (Fig. 1.34). This subtype is characterized by a dense chronic inflammatory lymphoplasmacytic background, in which isolated, scattered adipocytes are embedded. Lymphoid follicles may be found. The finding of atypical stromal cells with hyperchromatic nuclei and multinucleated giant cells represents an important diagnostic tool (Fig. 1.35a–c).
D. *Spindle cell subtype* (Fig. 1.36). In this subtype, spindle cells with large atypical nuclei, embedded in a dense fibrous or fibro-myxoid background, are the most abundant component. Stromal cells show markedly atypical nuclei. Adipocytes are often more focal and lipoblasts are scattered and patchy, so the adipocytic nature of the tumor may be overlooked, particularly in needle biopsies (Fig. 1.37). This variant is now considered to be the atypical variant of spindle cell lipoma.

Immunohistochemistry Nuclear immunoreactivity for MDM2 and/or CDK4 can be seen in the adipocytic (Fig. 1.38a, b), sclerosing (Fig. 1.38c), and inflammatory (Fig. 1.38d) variants. Nevertheless, expression of these proteins is often lacking (FISH/CISH is much more sensitive). The spindle cell variant shows loss of Rb, and is thus related to spindle cell lipoma.

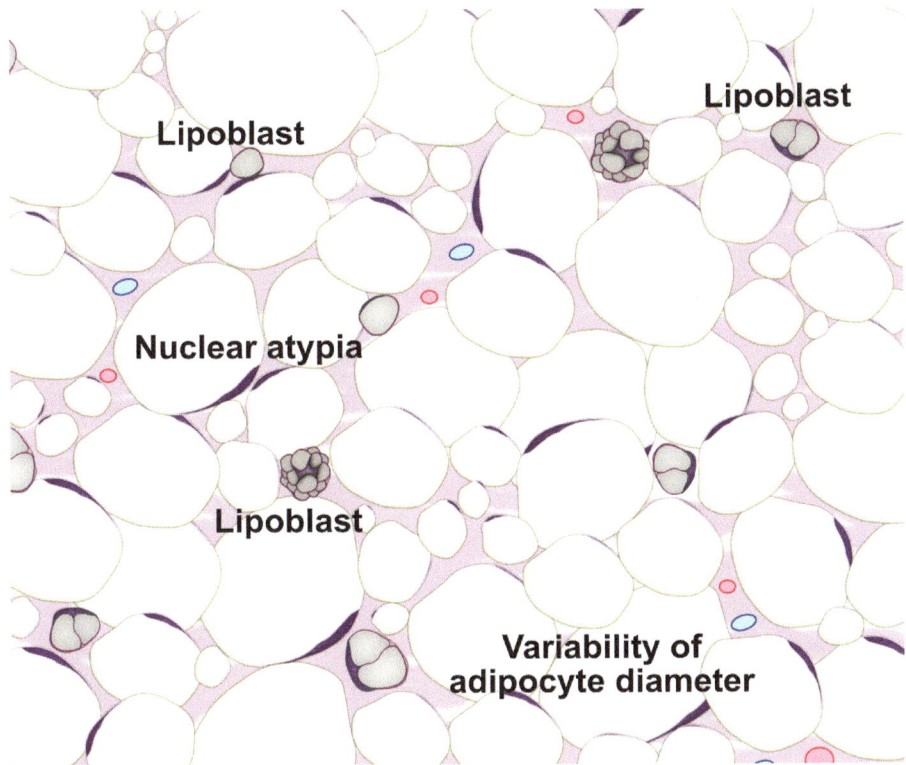

Fig. 1.30 Schematic representation of lipoma-like ALT/WDLPS

Molecular Genetics (Fig. 1.39a, b) Amplification of the *MDM2/CDK4* gene is classically observed in the lipoma-like, sclerosing, and inflammatory subtypes. Deletion of 13q14 can be found in the spindle cell variant.

Prognosis The mortality rate of ALT/WDLPS is strictly related to the site of origin, ranging from 0% in the extremities, where complete surgical removal is obtainable, to >80% in tumors originating in the retroperitoneum. The latter relates to a high recurrence rate and risk of dedifferentiation. Pure ALT/WDLPS has no metastatic potential.

Differential Diagnosis
1. *Benign lipoma:* the finding of marked variation in size and shape of adipocytes always lays stress on the hypothesis of an ALT/WDLPS. Lipoblasts, when present, are another sign in favor of ALT/WDLPS, but their absence has no significance. The presence of cytological atypia, both in adipocytes and in stromal cells, is helpful in establishing a diagnosis of malignancy.

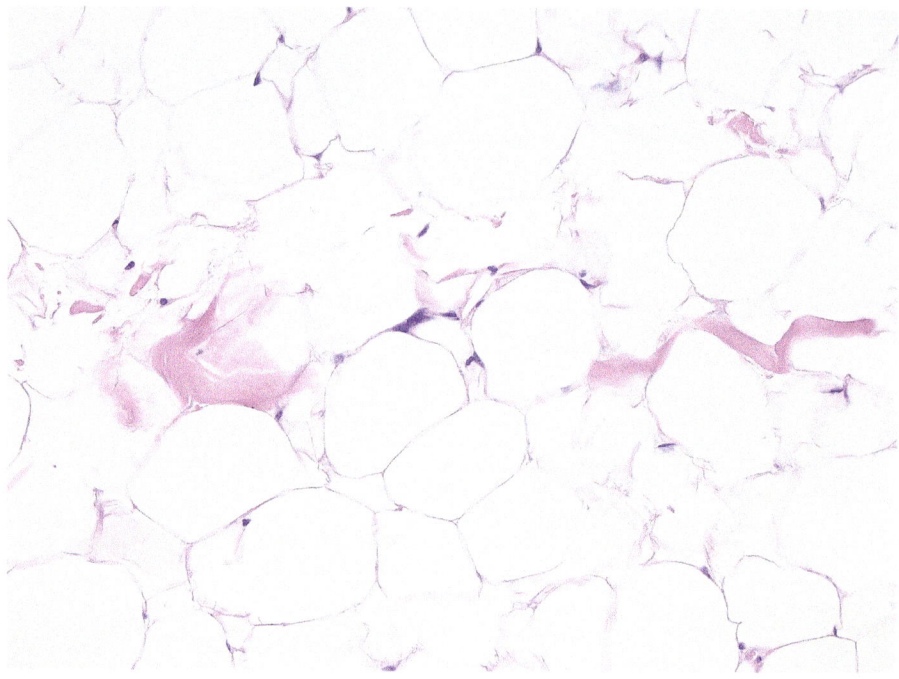

Fig. 1.31 Lipoma-like ALT/WDLPS (HE-stained section), showing hyperchromatic nuclei

2. *Idiopathic retroperitoneal fibrosis:* the presence of atypical stromal cells and immunoreactivity for MDM2, associated with *MDM2* gene amplification evidenced by FISH or CISH, are helpful for the diagnosis of WDLPS, sclerosing subtype.
3. *Inflammatory myofibroblastic tumor (IMT):* the absence of reactivity for smooth muscle actin, desmin and ALK protein, typical of myofibroblasts in IMT, and expression/amplification of *MDM2*, favor the diagnosis of WDLPS, inflammatory subtype.
4. *Massive localized lymphedema:* a pseudoneoplasm occurring in morbid obese patients. Prominent edema and fibrosis are seen, with septa encasing fat lobules, as well as numerous lymph and blood vessels and atypical spindle cells.

Dedifferentiated Liposarcoma (DDLPS)

Definition Malignant adipocytic neoplasm showing progression from well-differentiated liposarcoma to a non-lipogenic sarcoma of variable histological grade and outlook. From a practical point of view, the diagnosis of DDLPS should be considered in many sarcomas with different phenotypes.

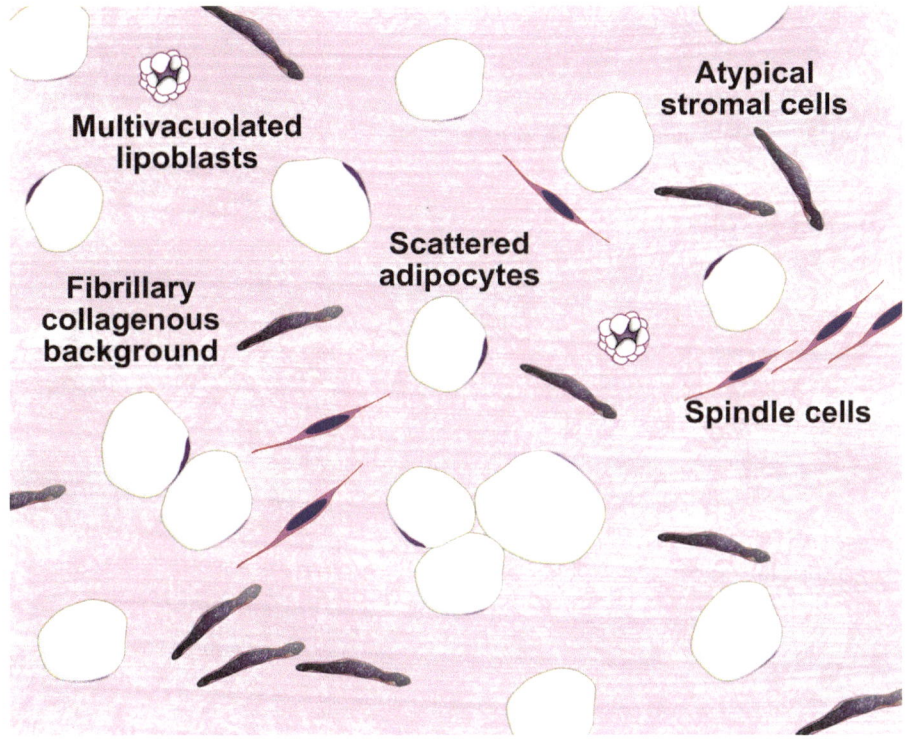

Fig. 1.32 Schematic representation of WDLPS, sclerosing subtype

Age at Presentation Adults to elderly, >40 years.

Gender Men more affected than women.

Localization Deep retroperitoneum (80%) > spermatic cord >limbs >trunk > mediastinum. Always deep.

Clinical Course It depends on the site of origin of the neoplasm and on the extent of surgical resection.

Macroscopy (Fig. 1.40) Large multinodular mass, yellow in color with firm gray areas. A firm gray nodule may be found in the background of yellow fatty nodules.

Microscopy The typical diagnostic feature of DDLPS is the abrupt transition from a well-differentiated lipoma-like liposarcoma to a high-grade non-lipogenic

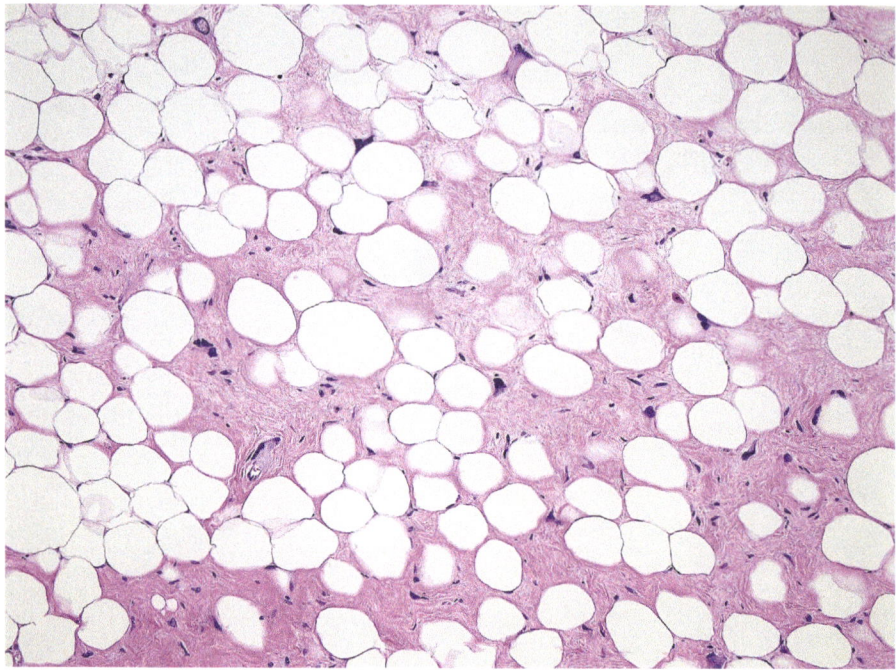

Fig. 1.33 Recurring retroperitoneal ALT/WDLPS, sclerosing type, from a 62-year-old male (HE-stained section)

spindle/pleomorphic sarcoma. The non-lipogenic component may be of variable grade and outlook, but often shows an aspecific spindle to pleomorphic sarcoma. Foci of heterologous differentiation may be present, including myogenic (rhabdomyoblastic or leiomyoid) (Fig. 1.41), osteo- (osteosarcomatous) (Fig. 1.42a, b), chondroid, angiosarcomatous, and meningothelial differentiation (Figs. 1.43 and 1.44a–c). Given the frequent localization in the retroperitoneum, the well-differentiated component may be interpreted as "normal surrounding fat tissue, leading to wrong diagnoses based exclusively on the dedifferentiated component(s). The dedifferentiated component may rarely be characterized by spindle cells in a fibrous background, with low-grade features (Figs. 1.45, 1.46, and 1.47a–d). In rare cases, the two components may appear intermingled, giving rise to scattered adipocytes in a background of high-grade (Fig. 1.48) spindle cell sarcoma. Some retroperitoneal tumors show a prominent neutrophilic infiltrate and correspond to the previously called inflammatory variant of malignant fibrous histiocytoma (MFH) (Fig. 1.49a–c). Rare tumors show a "homologous" lipoblastic (pleomorphic liposarcoma-like) picture. Not rarely, the well-differentiated component may be completely lacking, not only – due to sampling errors – in small biopsies but also in resections.

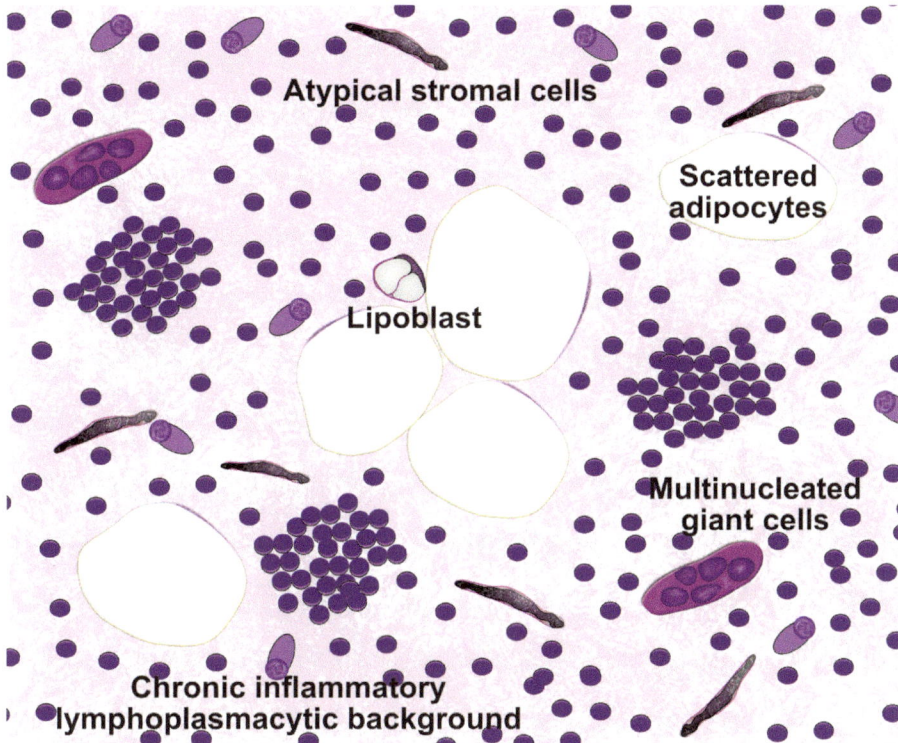

Fig. 1.34 Schematic representation of ALT/WDLPS, inflammatory subtype

Immunohistochemistry Both components of DDLPS show a strong nuclear immunoreactivity for MDM2 and CDK4, which is often more diffuse in the non-lipogenic component (reactivity is higher (stronger and more diffuse) than in WDLPS).

Caveat Nuclear immunoreactivity for MDM2 is often found in monocytes/macrophages, but there is no amplification of the gene (FISH negative).

Molecular Genetics Ring chromosomes or long markers, consisting of amplified 12q14–15 sequences, contain multiple copies of *MDM2/CDK4*. In situ hybridization shows amplification of *MDM2/CDK4*. Other genetic changes include 6q23 and 1p32 (*JUN*) co-amplifications.

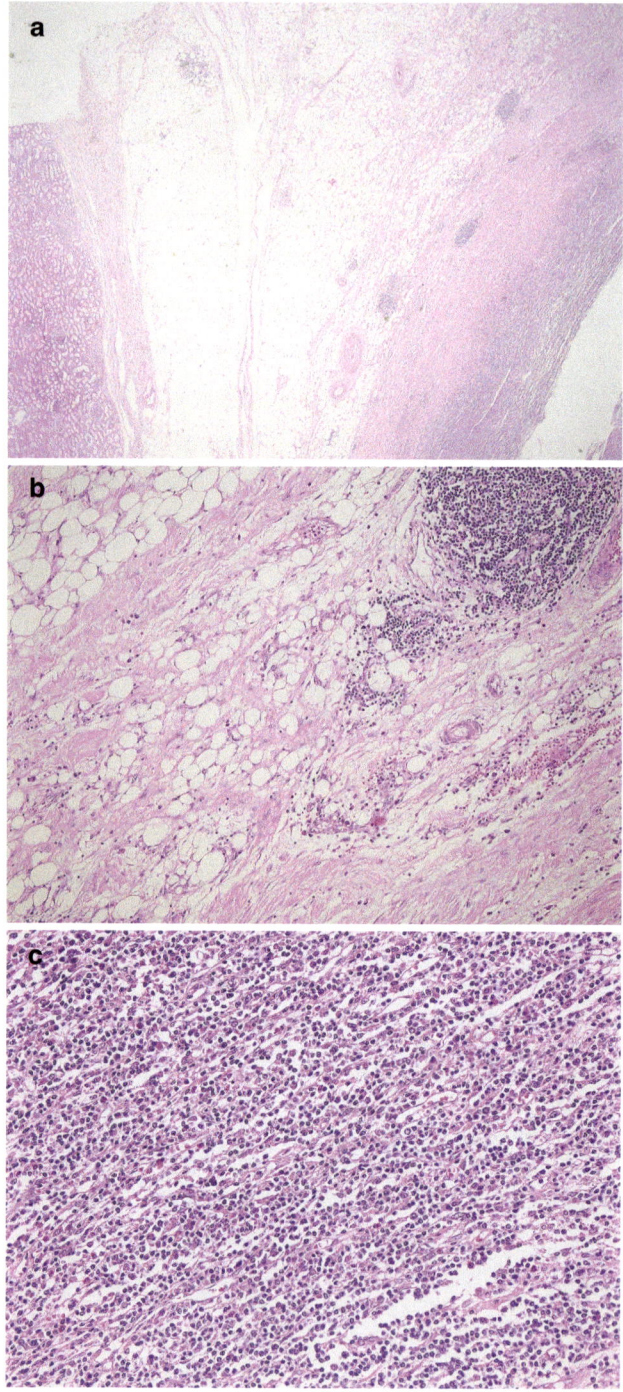

Fig. 1.35 Retroperitoneal ALT/WDLPS, inflammatory type, from a 67-year-old male at different power fields (**a–c**) (HE-stained section)

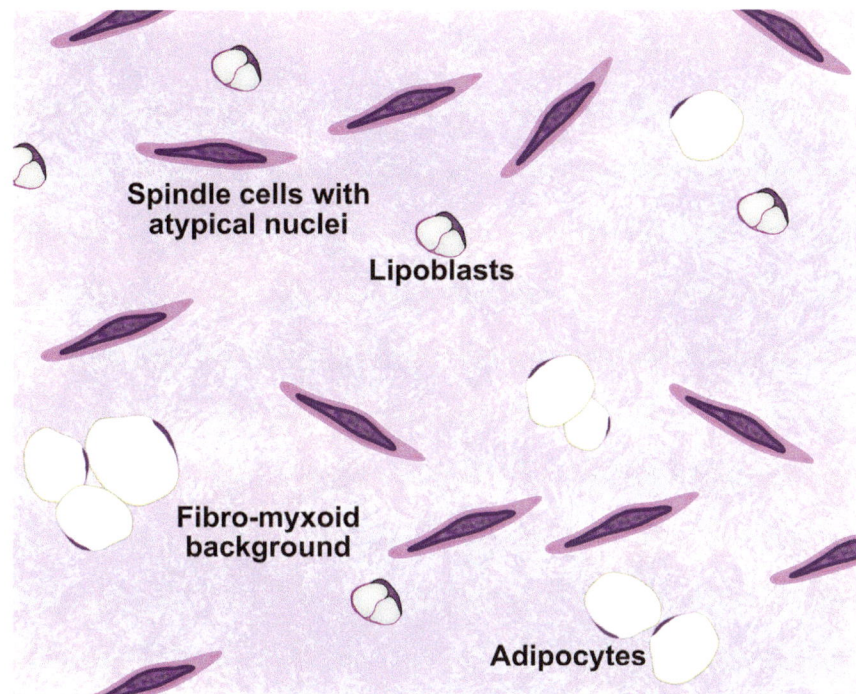

Fig. 1.36 Schematic representation of ALT/WDLPS, spindle cell subtype

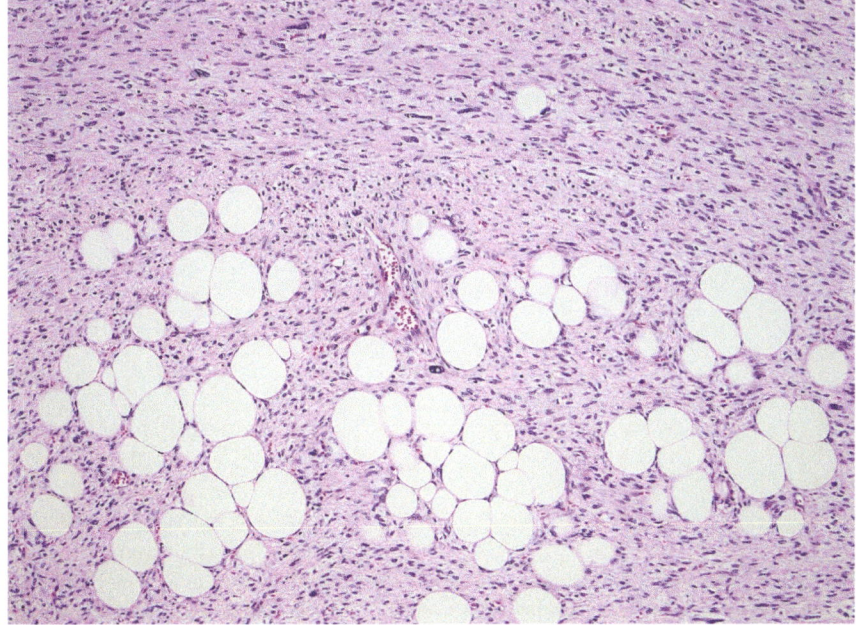

Fig. 1.37 Orbital ALT/WDLPS, spindle cell type, from a 20-year-old male (HE-stained section)

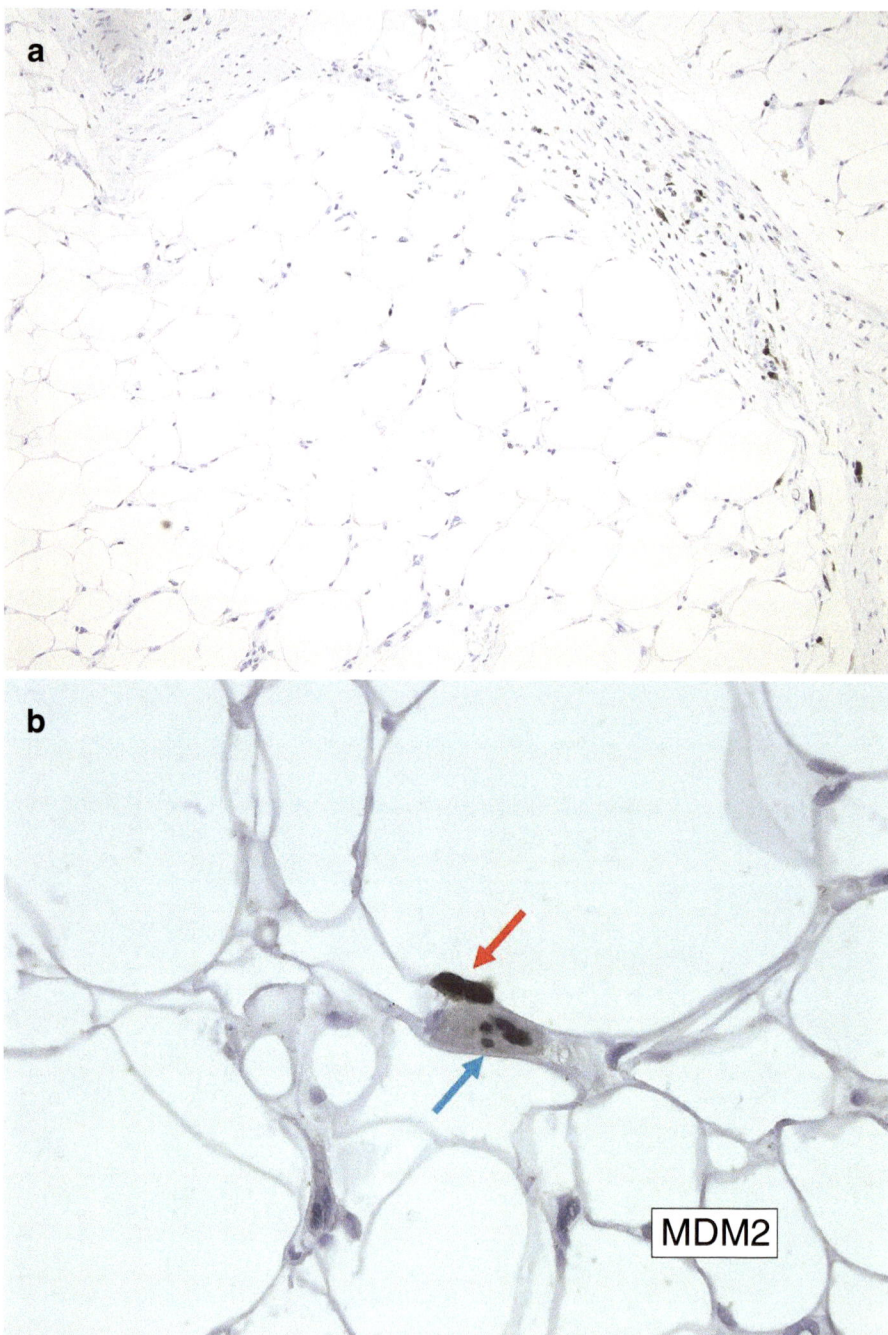

Fig. 1.38 MDM2 immunoreactivity of ALT/WDLPS, lipoma-like type, at low- magnification (**a**) and at high-power field. Red arrow indicates nuclear positivity in a tumor cell and blue arrow in a macrophage (**b**), sclerosing type (**c**), and inflammatory subtype (**d**)

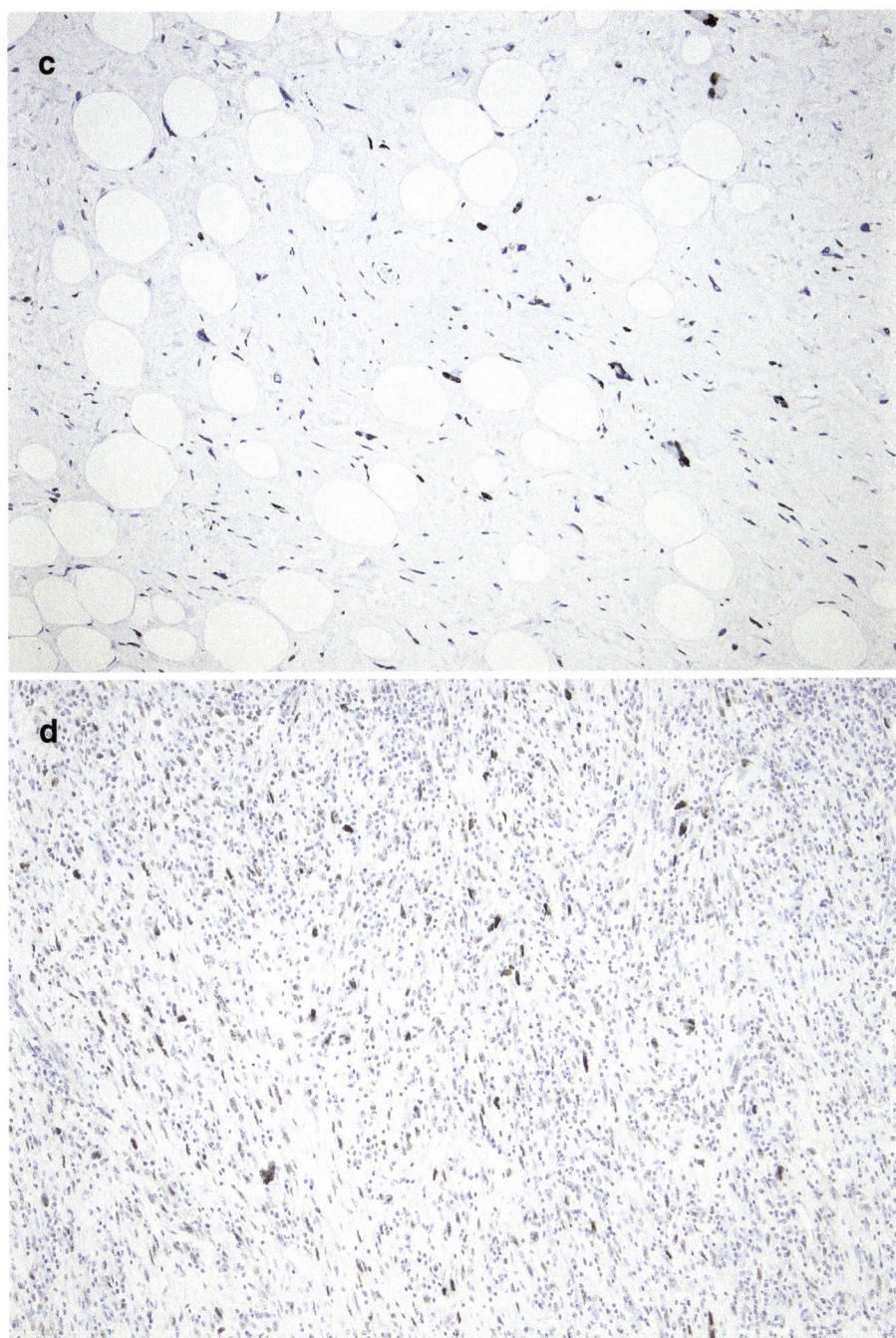

Fig. 1.38 (continued)

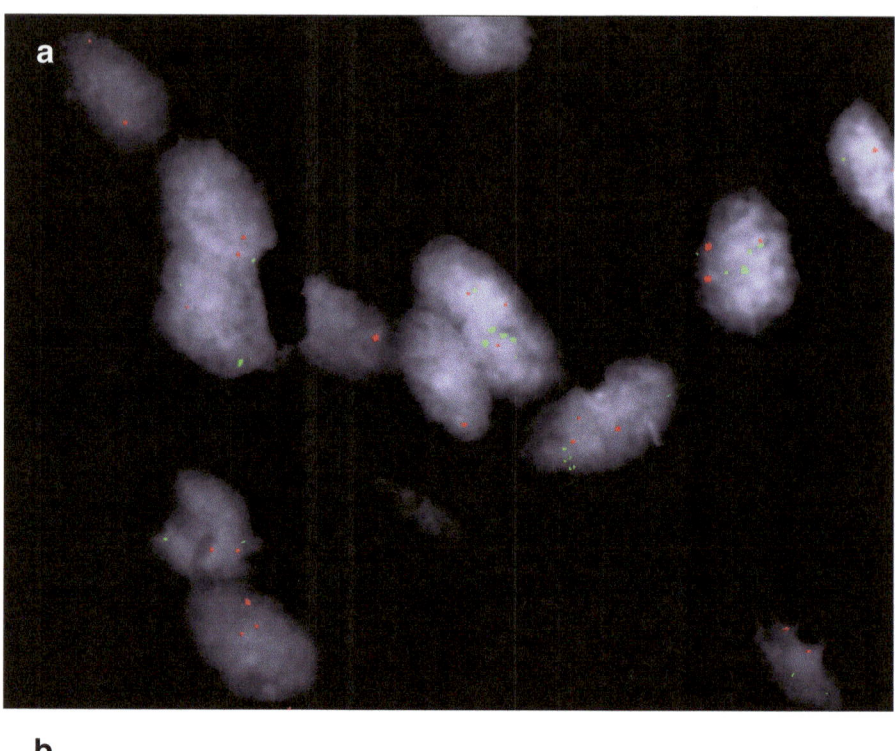

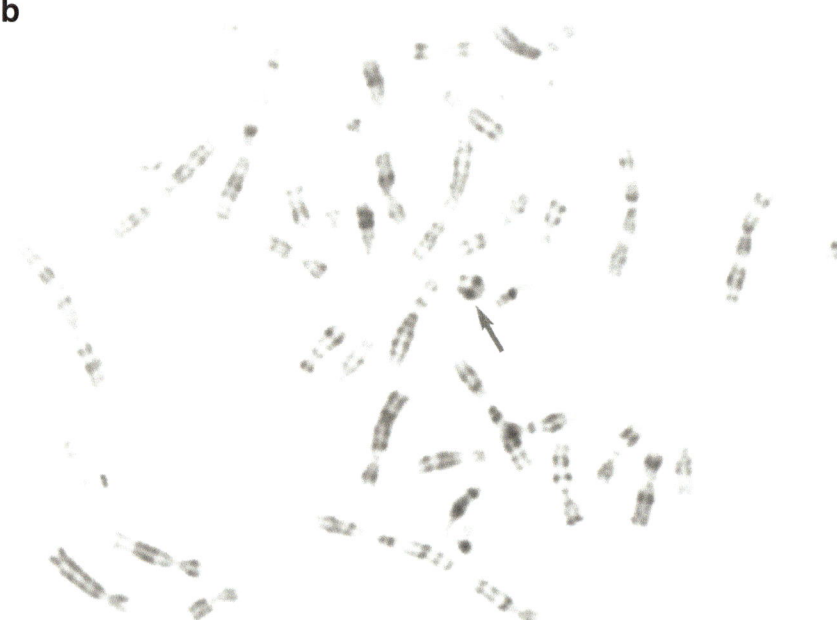

Fig. 1.39 Amplification of *MDM2* gene: in green, MDM2/12q14-BIO probe; in red, *CDK4*/12q13-DIG probe (**a**); cytogenetic map with long markers and rings (arrow) (**b**)

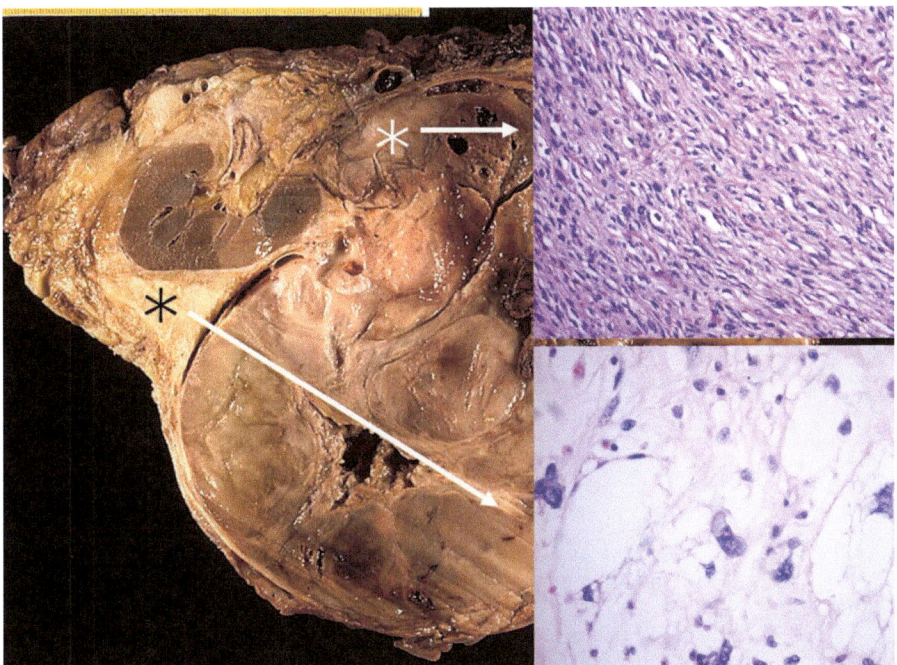

Fig. 1.40 Correlation between the macroscopic and histologic (HE-stained) pictures in a retroperitoneal dedifferentiated liposarcoma with a diameter of 35 cm, from a 66-year-old male

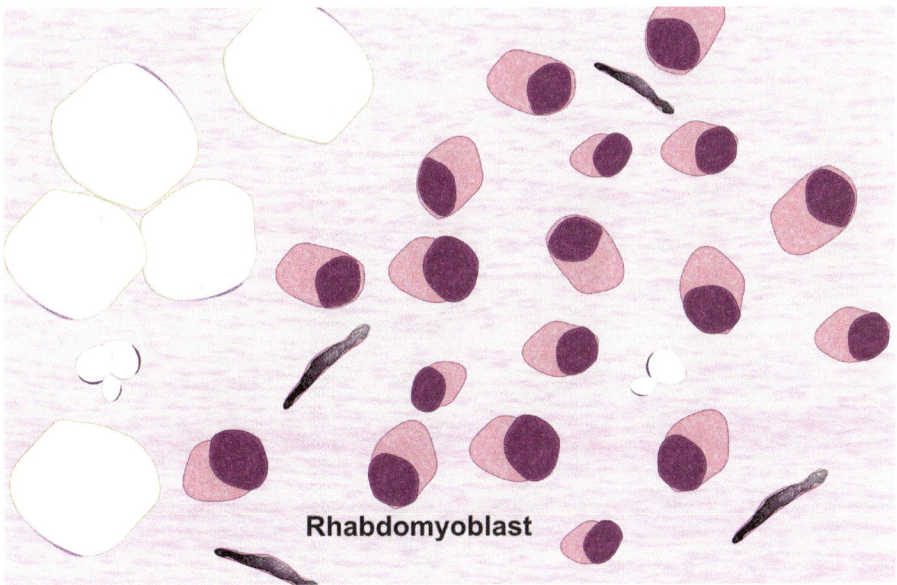

Fig. 1.41 Schematic representation of DDLPS with rhabdomyoblastic differentiation

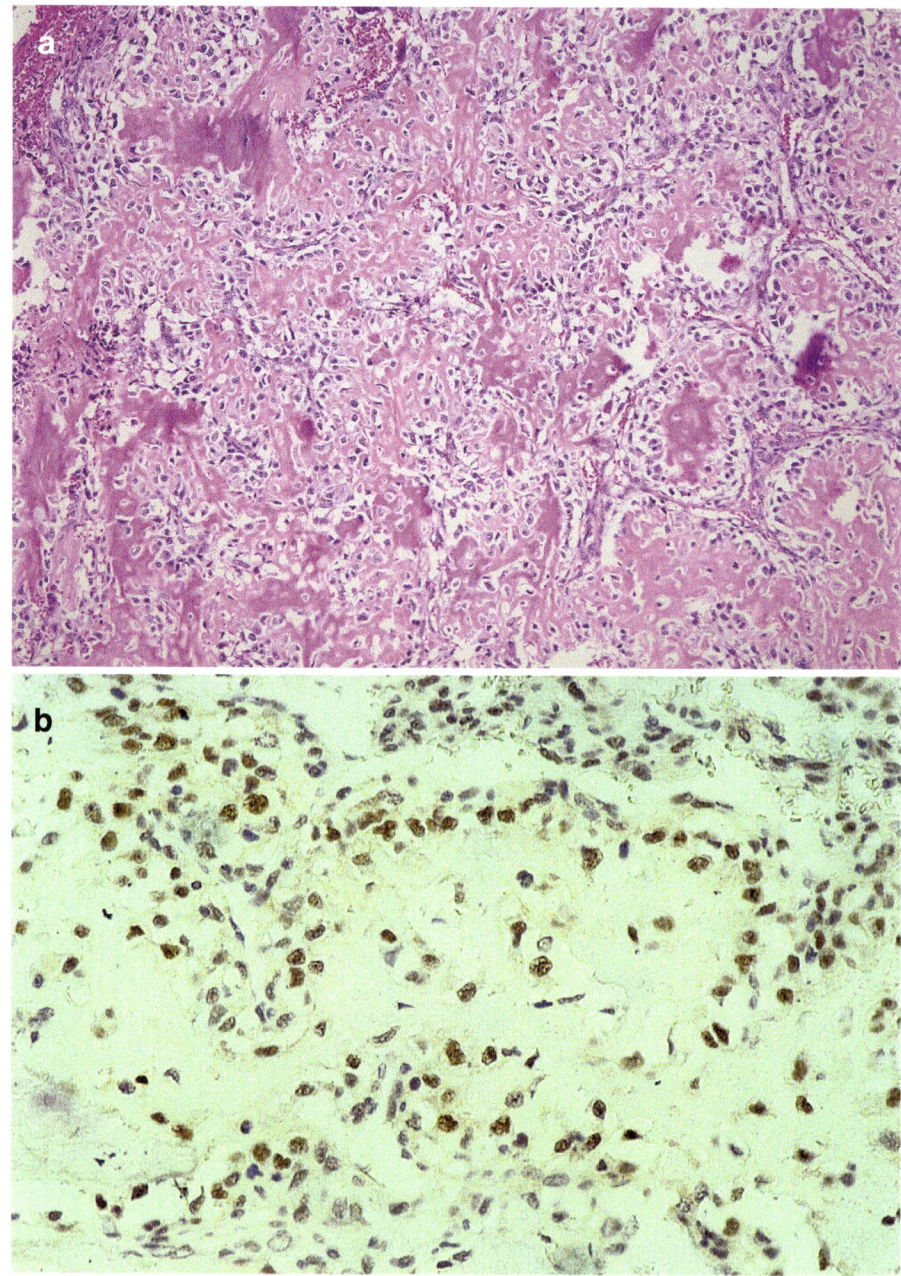

Fig. 1.42 DDLPS with bone formation (**a**: HE-stained sections; **b**: immunohistochemistry for MDM2)

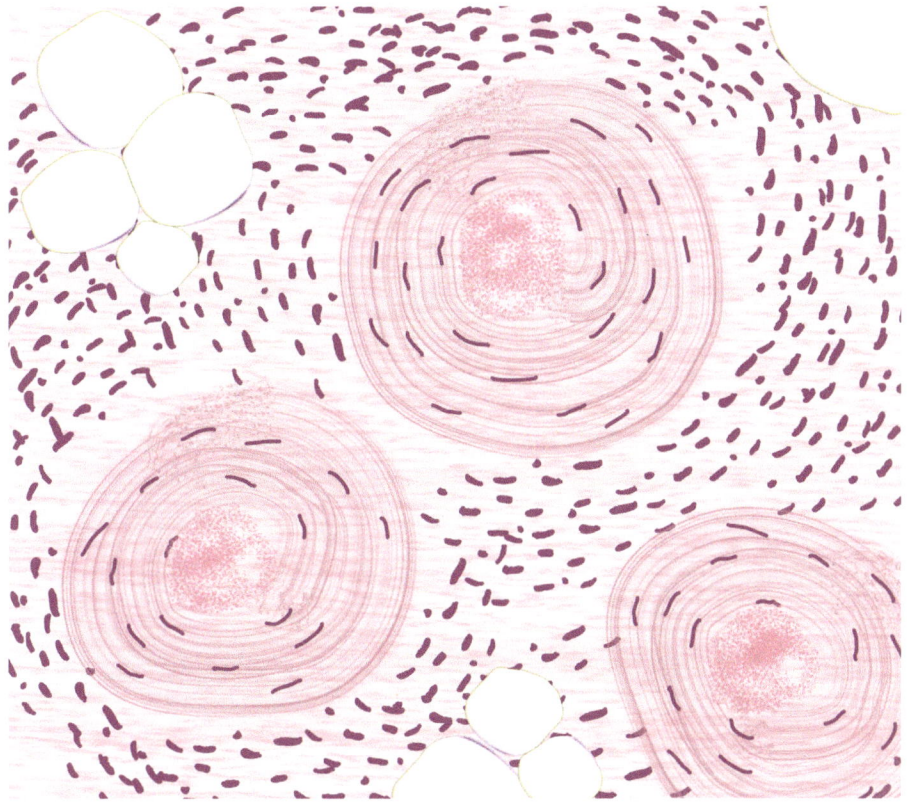

Fig. 1.43 DDLPS with DDLPS with meningothelial whorls

Differential Diagnosis
1. *Pleomorphic leiomyosarcoma* may be differentiated by the expression of desmin, smooth muscle actin, and h-Caldesmon in the absence of obvious *MDM2* amplification.
2. *Gastrointestinal stromal tumor* (GIST) may be differentiated by the expression of DOG1 and CD117.
3. *Sarcomatoid carcinoma* may be excluded by the absence of expression of cytokeratins and epithelial membrane antigen (EMA) in the presence of *MDM2* amplification.

From a practical point of view, FISH for MDM2 is mandatory in every case of undifferentiated sarcoma, in order to not avoid a correct diagnosis of DDLPS.

Prognosis DDLPS, in spite of the often high morphological grade, is less aggressive and has a better prognosis as compared to other pleomorphic sarcomas. The metastatic rate is 15–30%, whereas the time to relapse is strictly related to the extent

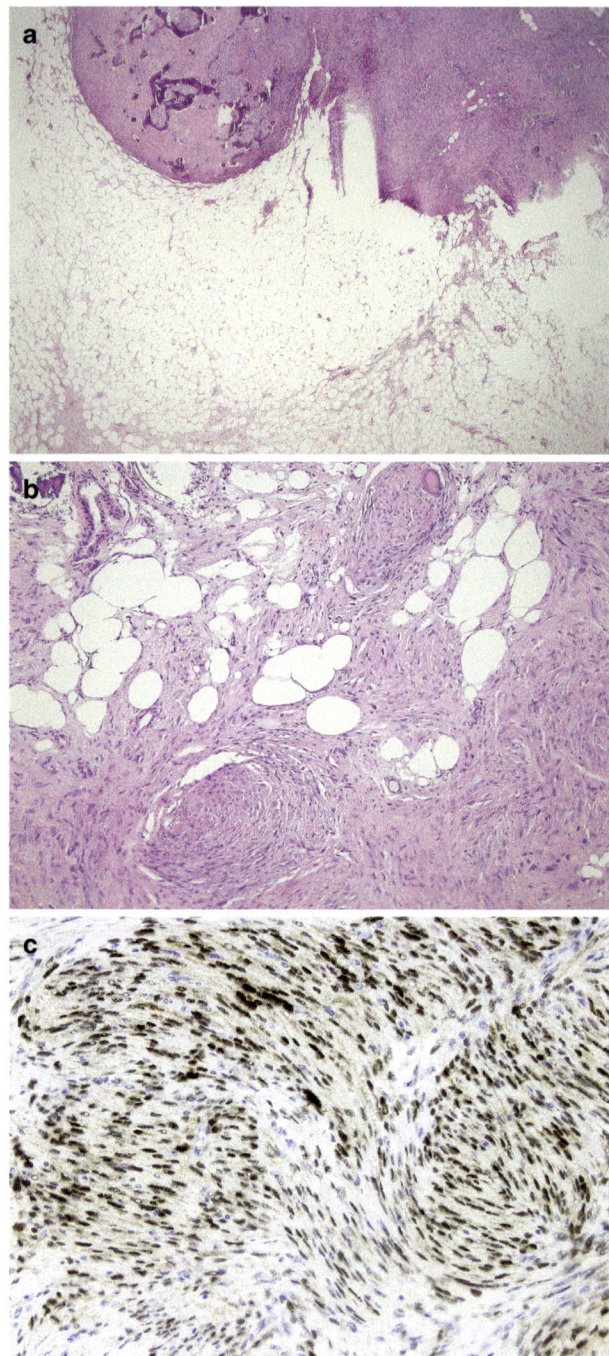

Fig. 1.44 Retroperitoneal DDLPS with meningothelial whorls and bone differentiation from a 54-year-old female at low-power (**a**) and high-power field (**b**) of magnification (HE-stained sections) and immunohistochemistry for MDM2 (**c**)

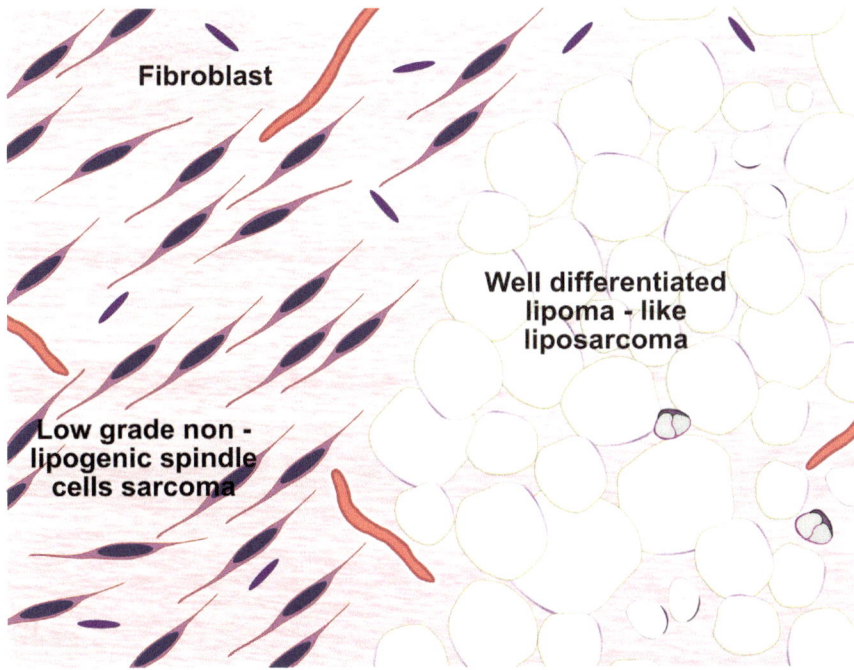

Fig. 1.45 Schematic representation of low-grade DDLPS

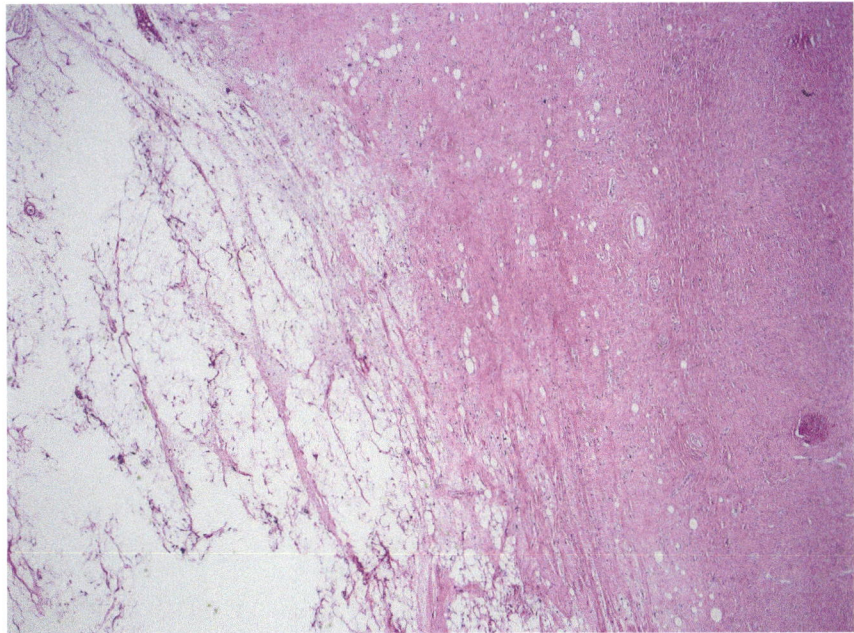

Fig. 1.46 Panoramic view of retroperitoneal low-grade DDLPS from a 58-year-old female (HE-stained sections)

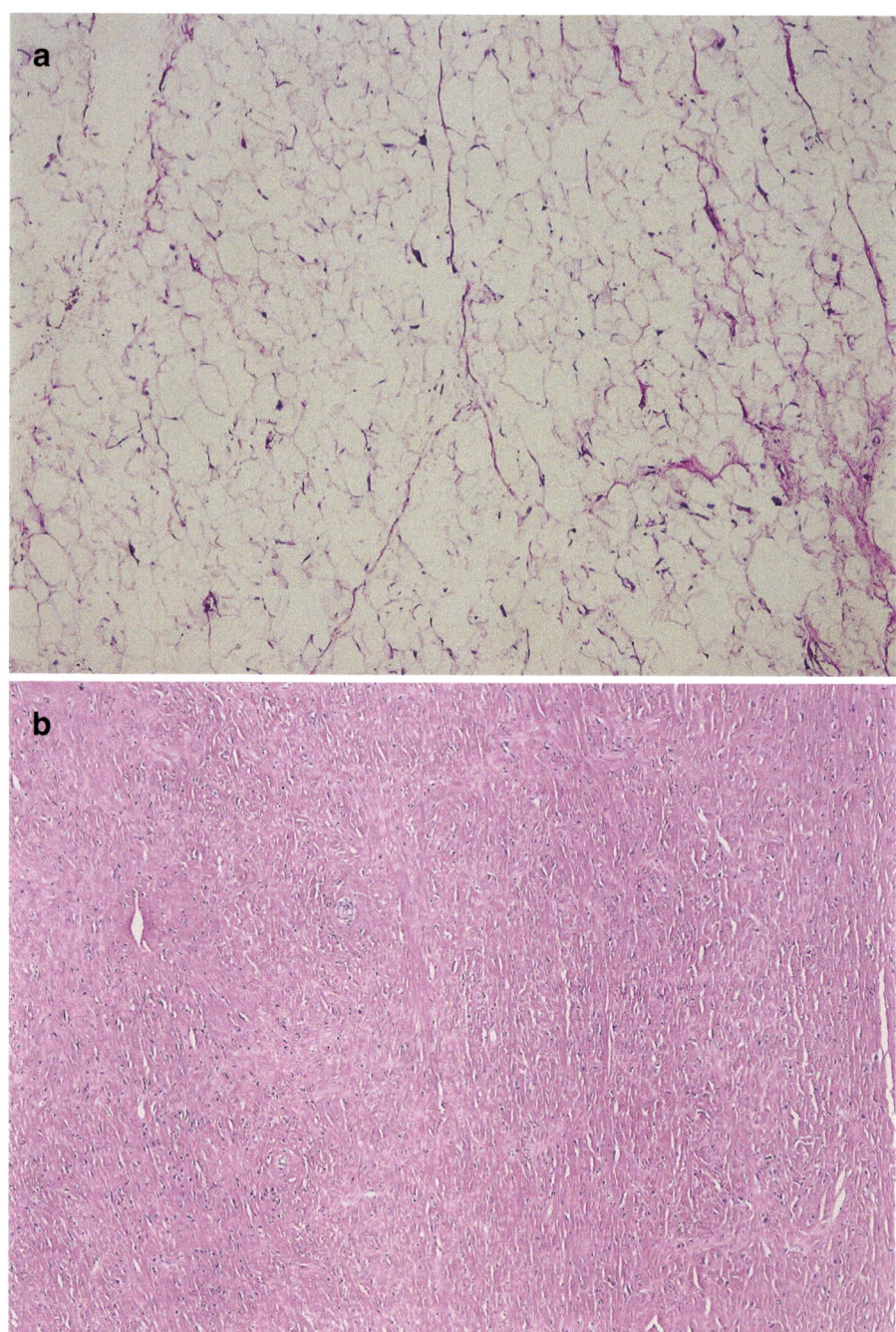

Fig. 1.47 Higher magnification of different histological patterns (HE-stained sections) (**a, b**) and MDM2 (**c, d**) expressions of the retroperitoneal low-grade DDLPS from a 58-year-old female mentioned in Fig. 1.46

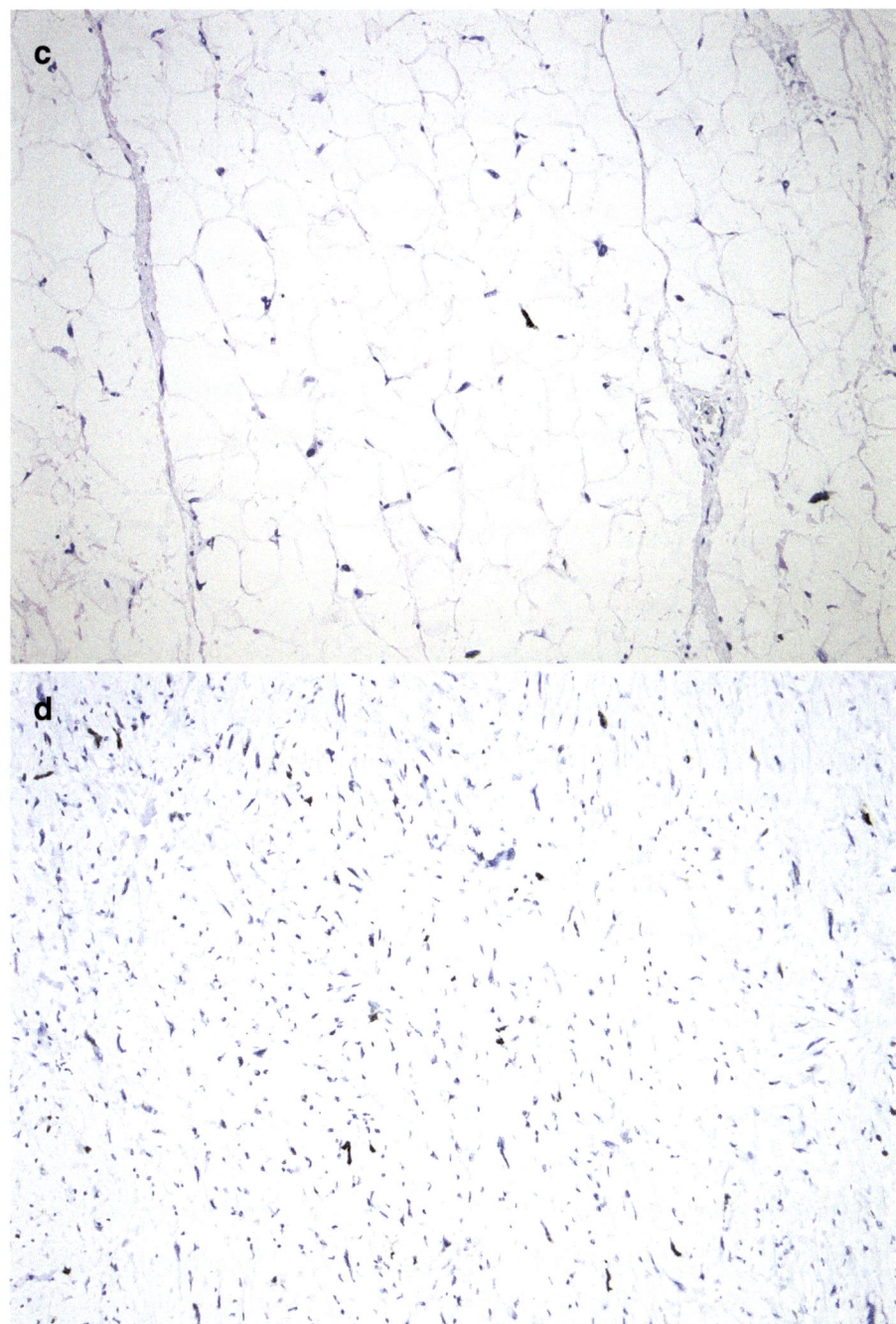

Fig. 1.47 (continued)

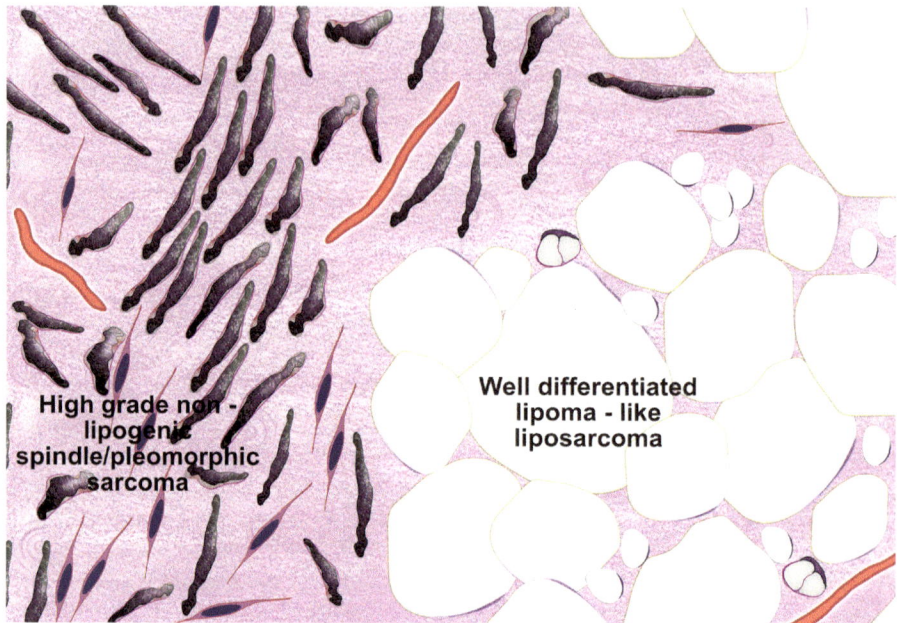

Fig. 1.48 Schematic representation of high-grade DDLPS

of surgical resection. High risk for recurrence is the case in the retroperitoneum. Whether the grade and outlook of the dedifferentiated part influence the prognosis is still not fully clear, but more recent studies tend to indicate that a high-grade tumor is more aggressive.

Myxoid/High-Grade Myxoid (Round Cell) Liposarcoma

Definition It is the second most frequent subtype of LPS, accounting for one-third of all liposarcomas. A morphologic continuum is seen between pure myxoid and pure round cell types. The term high-grade myxoid liposarcoma is now used to indicate the latter type since a round cell phenotype is not always seen.

Age at Presentation It is the commonest LPS of young adults (30–40 years).

Gender Equal gender distribution.

Localization Lower limbs (thigh). Extremely rare in the retroperitoneum.

Clinical Course A nodule in the thigh is the typical presentation. The neoplasm may be responsible for unusual metastatic sites: retroperitoneum, axilla, pleura, bone.

Fig. 1.49 DDLPS with 'inflammatory MFH-like' picture from the left psoas of a 74-year-old female, at different power fields (HE stain) (**a, b**) with the immunohistochemistry for MDM2 (**c**)

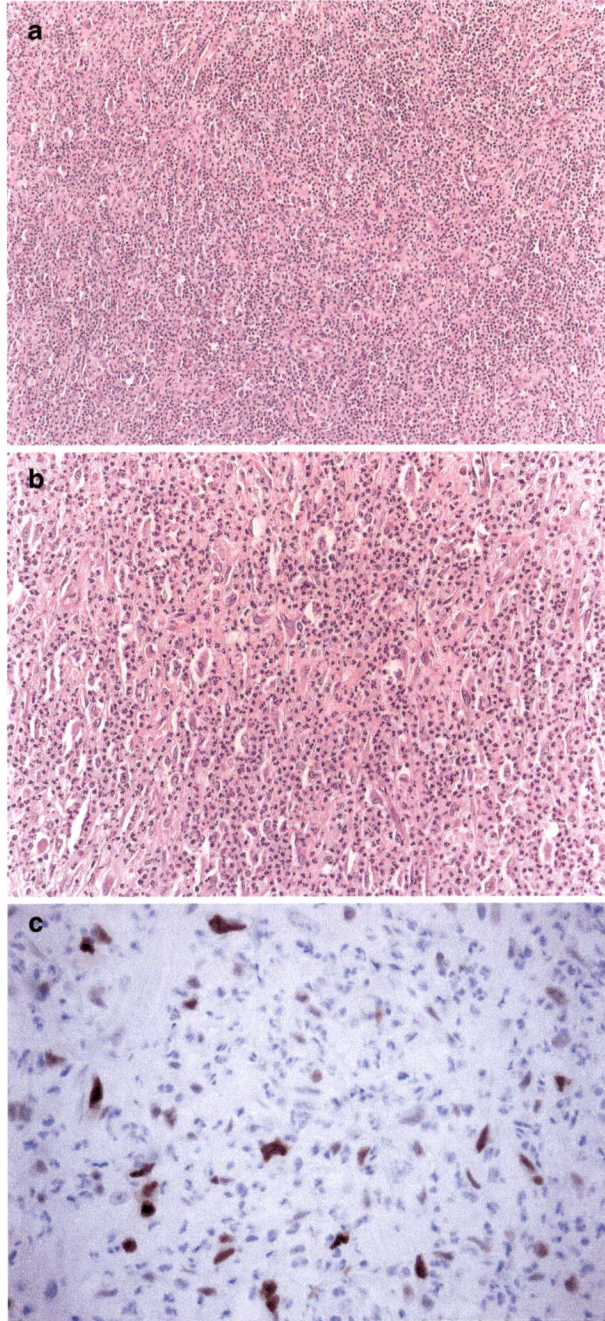

Macroscopy Well circumscribed nodule or multinodular mass, of gelatinous consistency. Fleshy areas may be present.

Microscopy Morphologic continuum from pure myxoid to high-grade pure round cell component. Atypia may be minimal or absent. A) Myxoid component (Fig. 1.50): hypocellular areas; myxoid bluish background (Fig. 1.51); prominent plexiform thin chicken-wire/crow's feet capillary network; mucin pools (lymphangioma-like, pulmonary edema-like) (Figs. 1.52 and 1.53a, b); bland stellate/spindle cells; univacuolated lipoblasts around vessels or at the periphery of the neoplasm. B) High grade (round cell) component (Fig. 1.54): hypercellular areas; round cells with scant cytoplasm and round nuclei with small nucleoli; round cells tend to aggregate around vessels; adipocytic differentiation often absent. The finding of hypercellular areas, existing of round or rarely spindle cells, in more than 5% of the tumor is indicative of a high-grade myxoid (round cell) LPS (Fig. 1.55).

Immunohistochemistry Not contributive.

Molecular Genetics 95% of myxoid LPS carry the t(12;16)(q13;p11), *FUS/DDIT3* (CHOP) gene fusion. A rare variant shows a t(12;22) (*DDIT3/EWSR1*) gene fusion (Fig. 1.56a, b).

Prognosis About 12–25% of the tumors recur. The 5-year survival rate of pure myxoid LPS is 90% and goes down to about 25% when the high-grade round cell component represents more than 25% of the tumor.

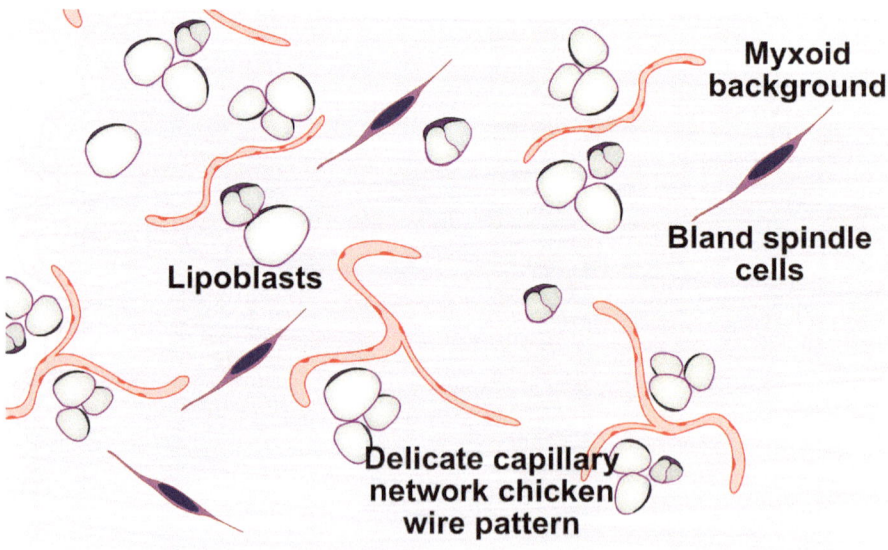

Fig. 1.50 Schematic representation of myxoid LPS

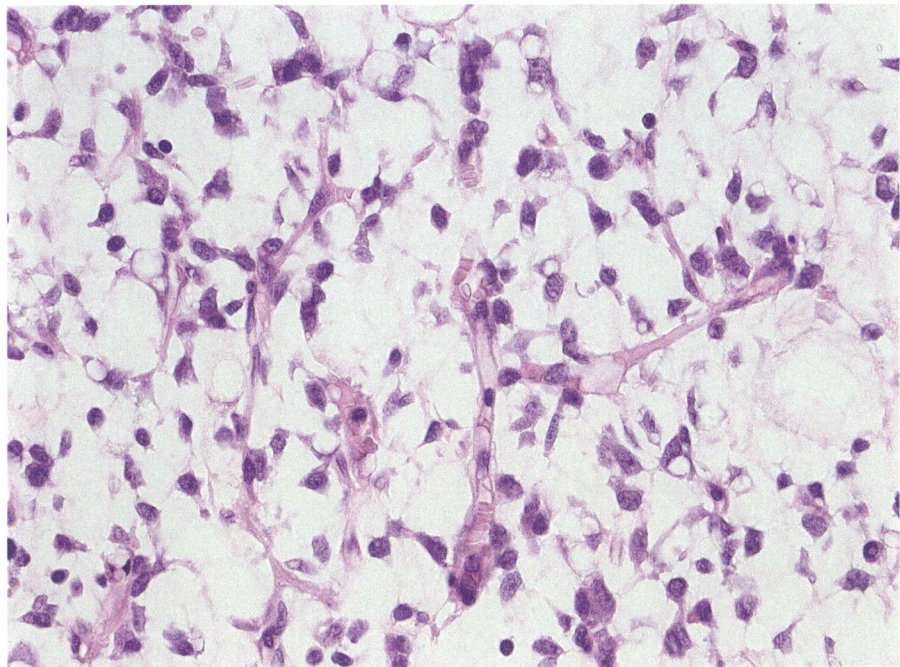

Fig. 1.51 Myxoid LPS (HE-stained sections)

Pleomorphic Liposarcoma (PLPS) (Fig. 1.57)

Definition Rare aggressive subtype of LPS, accounting for 5% of all LPS, characterized by the presence of large, highly atypical lipoblasts.

Age at Presentation From adults to elderly people (peaks in the seventh decade).

Gender Men slightly more affected.

Localization Extremities (lower limbs, thigh) > trunk > mediastinum > retroperitoneum.

Clinical Presentation Well-demarcated deep mass, rapidly enlarging.

Macroscopy Fleshy on cut surface, with hemorrhagic and necrotic areas.

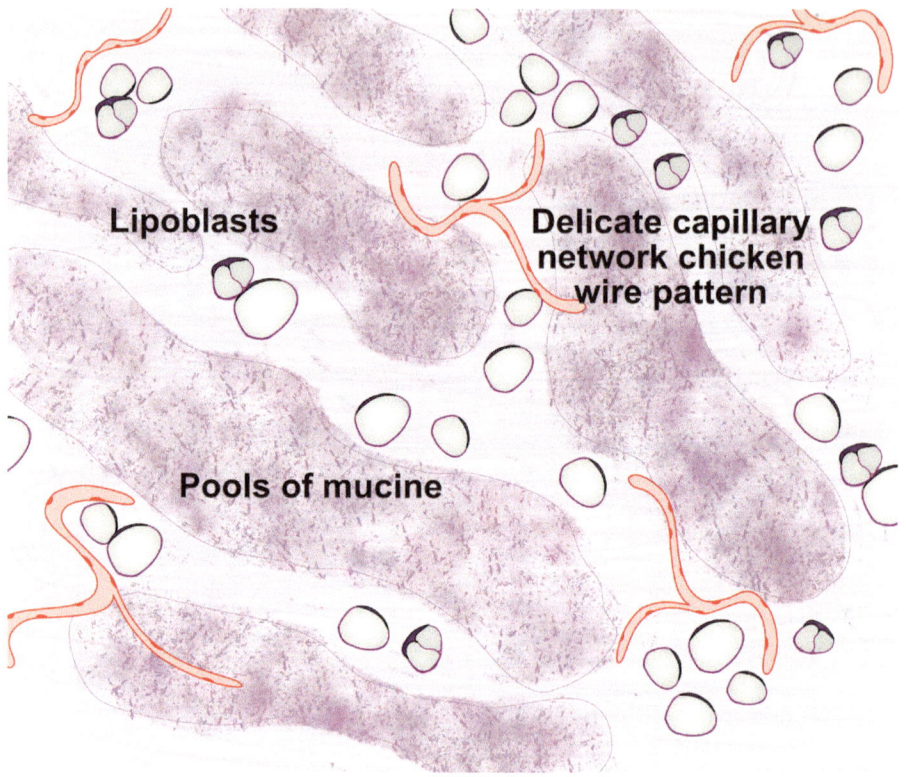

Fig. 1.52 Schematic representation of pulmonary edema-like myxoid LPS

Microscopy Large atypical pleomorphic multivacuolated lipoblasts in the background of a high-grade sarcoma. Cytological atypia is very prominent (Fig. 1.58a, b), lipoblasts can be focal, requiring an accurate sampling. High mitotic activity. Frequent foci of intratumoral necrosis. Foci of epithelioid differentiation of tumor cells may be present (Fig. 1.59).

Immunohistochemistry Not contributive, but there is no immunostaining for MDM2. The epithelioid variant may express keratin or Melan-A.

Molecular Genetics Non-consistent complex genetic changes.

Prognosis High-grade sarcoma. Overall 5-year survival rate: 60%. Metastatic rate 30–40%. Rare superficial cases occurring in the skin show a more favorable prognosis.

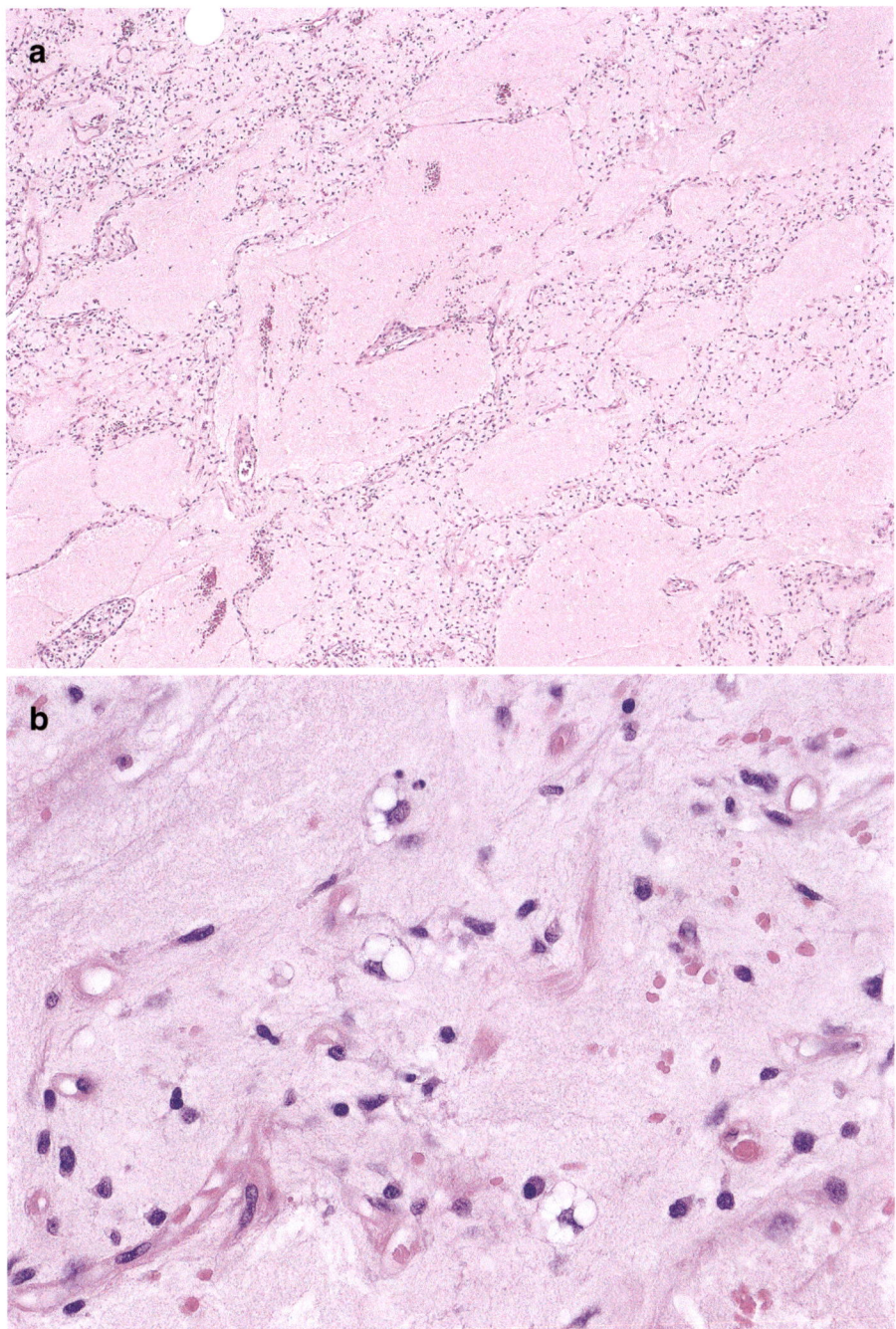

Fig. 1.53 Pulmonary edema-like areas in myxoid LPS in the upper leg, from a palpable mass after trauma, of a 52 year-old male at low-power (**a**) and high-power field (**b**) of magnification (HE-stained sections)

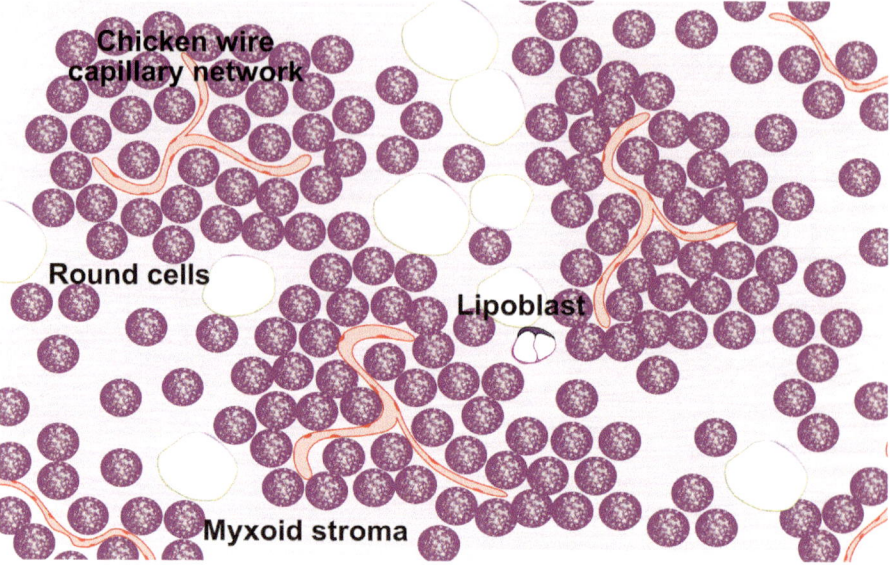

Fig. 1.54 Schematic representation of high-grade (round cell) myxoid LPS

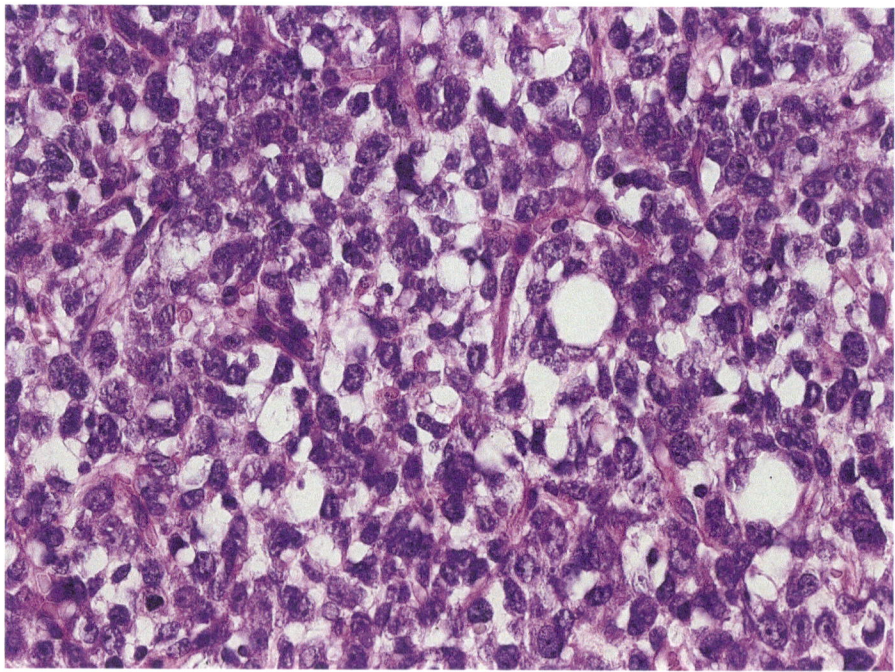

Fig. 1.55 High-grade myxoid round cell LPS (HE-stained section)

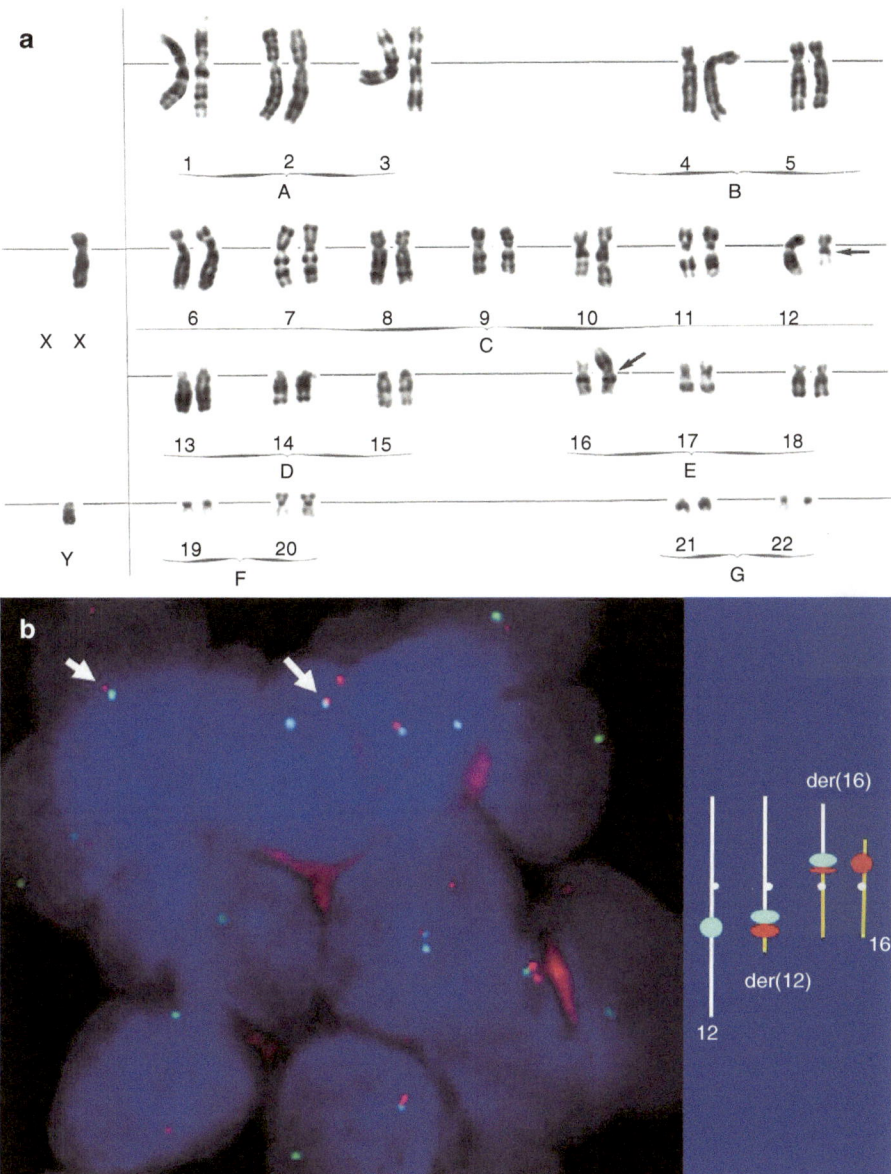

Fig. 1.56 Cytogenetic map (**a**) of 46,XY, t(12;16)(q13;p11) FUS-DDIT3 fusion gene in the myxoid round cell LPS; FISH (**b**) and FISH bring-together approach (green: DDIT3/12q13-BIO probe; red: FUS/16p11-DIG probe)

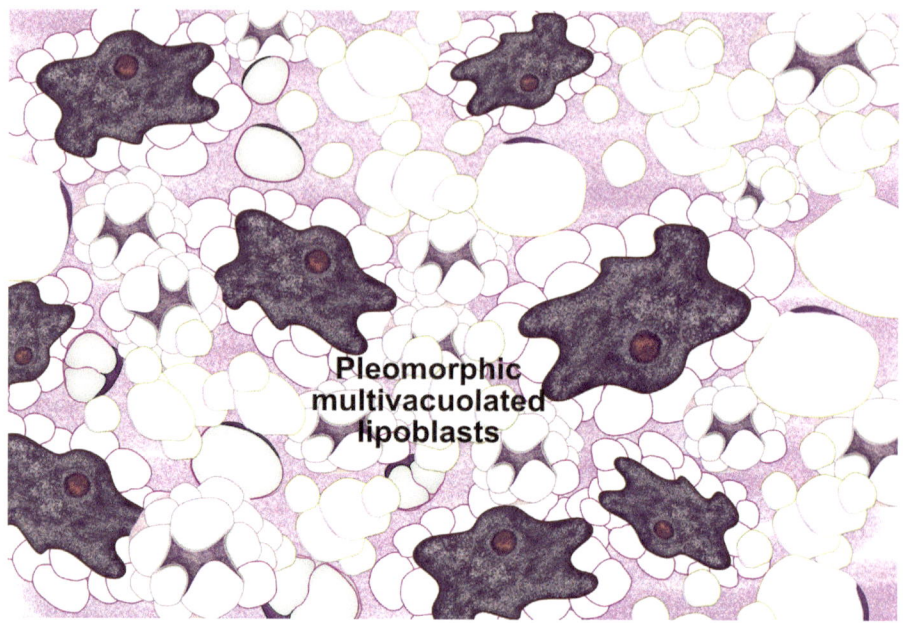

Fig. 1.57 Schematic representation of pleomorphic liposarcoma

Differential Diagnosis

A. *DDLPS*: may be difficult to differentiate, mainly in needle biopsy, when the differentiated part of the tumor has not been sampled. Nuclear immunoreactivity of spindle cells and lipoblasts for MDM2 and CDK4 indicates DDLPS.

B. *Carcinoma*, particularly renal cell carcinoma (RCC) may enter in the DD with the epithelioid variant of PLPS. A strong and diffuse reactivity for keratin, in the absence of MDM2 expression, supports the diagnosis of carcinoma.

In the last WHO update on the classification of soft tissue tumors in 2020, an exceptionally rare subtype of liposarcoma has been included: the so-called "myxoid pleomorphic liposarcoma." This tumor occurs in young patients (10–20 years old), is mainly seen in the mediastinum, and is rarely seen in the thigh or head and neck region. It combines the histology of myxoid and pleomorphic liposarcoma and shows numerical chromosomal changes and inactivation of RB. This sarcoma seems to be very aggressive.

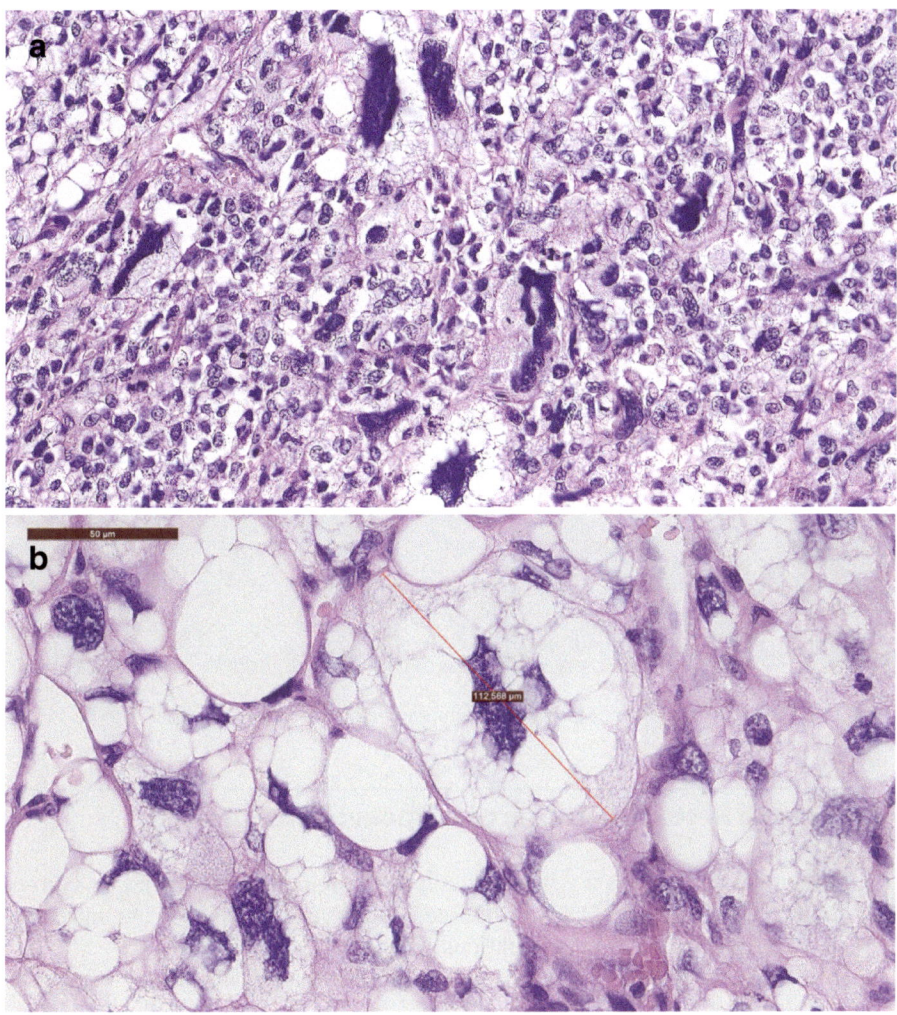

Fig. 1.58 Pleomorphic liposarcoma from the pectoralis major muscle in a 34-year-old male at low-power (a) and at high-power field (b) of magnification (HE-stained section)

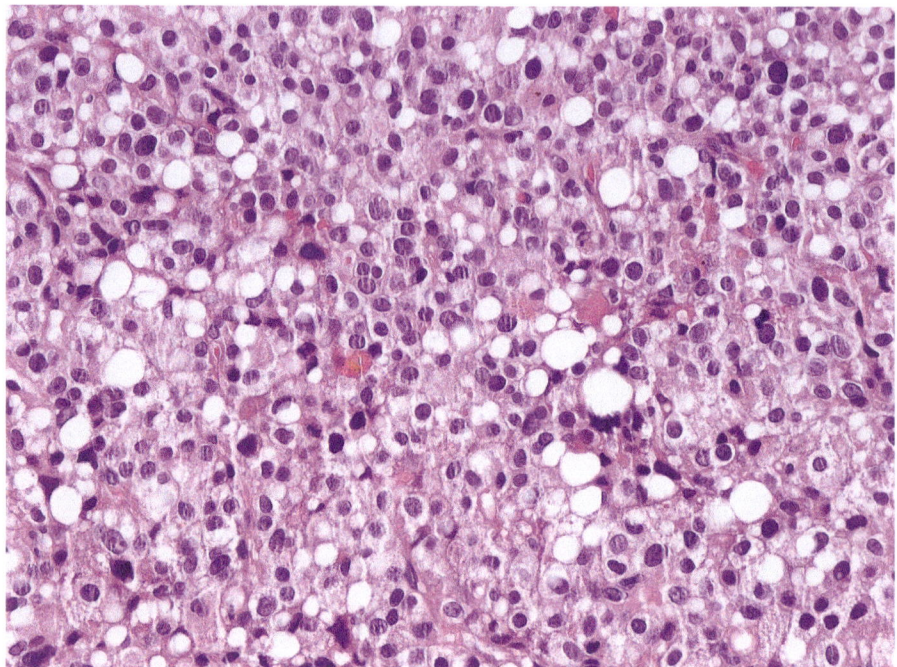

Fig. 1.59 Epithelioid variant of pleomorphic liposarcoma (HE-stained section)

Tricks for a Better Diagnosis of Adipocytic Tumors

1. Diagnosis of malignancy in many adipocytic tumors is not based on conventional malignancy criteria but is defined by the entity itself, making underdiagnosis of malignancy likely in entities such as ATL/WDLPS.
2. Deep first: deep lesions are more suspicious for malignancy. However, superficial location does NOT exclude a liposarcoma.
3. Infiltrative margins are NOT always a sign of aggressive behavior.
4. Well-differentiated adipocytic differentiation is NOT always a sign of benign tumor (see ALT/WDLPS).
5. The presence of lipoblasts is NOT always a sign of malignancy (see lipoblastoma/chondroid/spindle, pleomorphic lipoma).
6. The absence of lipoblasts does NOT exclude the diagnosis of liposarcoma.
7. Lipoblast-like cells may be encountered in non-tumoral reactive processes, including silicone granuloma of the breast.
8. The morphology of intratumoral vessels may help in the diagnosis of adipocytic tumors:
   (a) Thin S-shaped chicken-wire capillary vessels are typically found in myxoid LPS and in myxoid areas of lipoblastoma

   (b) Thick-walled vessels, lacking an elastica, are typically found in angiomyolipoma.

9. Hypereosinophilic collagen ropy fibers are typically observed in spindle cell/pleomorphic lipoma.

10. Markedly pleomorphic cells are not per se indicative of malignant adipocytic tumors (see pleomorphic lipoma).

11. Nuclear reactivity for MDM2 may be found in normal reactive macrophages, but amplification is lacking. Cytoplasmic MDM2 expression is of no significance.

12. The absence of immunoreactivity for MDM2 does not exclude the diagnosis of LPS, certainly in ATL/WDLPS. FISH (or CISH) is much more sensitive, revealing gene amplification even in cases with low or absent immunostaining for MDM2.

13. The diagnosis of DDLPS should be considered in any unclassifiable sarcoma, even in the absence of the well-differentiated adipocytic component. Consider the impact of sampling variability, when dealing with thin needle biopsies!

14. A prominent neural-like meningothelioma-like whorling pattern – often associated with mature bone – mainly in a sarcoma located in the retroperitoneum should raise the suspicion of DDLPS (go to FISH for MDM2).

15. The presence of capillaries with thrombi is typical of angiolipoma.

16. Apparently normal looking fat that surrounds a retroperitoneal tumor should be sampled in order to not miss a potential well-differentiated component of DDLPS.

17. Prominent variation in adipocyte size, associated with nuclear prominence and atypia of adipocytic and stromal cell nuclei, should always be suspicious for ALT/WDLPS.

18. Nuclear prominence and variation in size of adipocytes have no meaning in adipocytic tumors located in fingers.

19. When to go to FISH (or CISH) for *MDM2* in the differential diagnosis of well-differentiated fatty tumors?
   (a) Deep lesion
   (b) Size>10 cm in diameter
   (c) Age at presentation >50 years
   (d) Equivocal atypia
   (e) When located in retroperitoneum, abdomen, pelvis. Neck and upper shoulder regions also deserve more attention.
   (f) In the presence of worrisome radiological features.
   (g) In all cases with a prominent inflammatory infiltrate that obscures the morphology of tumor cells.

20. High grade is NOT always associated with bad prognosis (DDLPS is less aggressive than other pleomorphic sarcomas).

21. DDLPS may mimic many tumors, including osteosarcoma, GIST, seminoma, carcinoma, desmoid.

Essential Bibliography

1. Al Hmada Y, Schaefer I-M, Fletcher CDM. Hibernoma mimicking atypical lipomatous tumor: 64 cases of a morphologically distinct subset. Am J Surg Pathol. 2018;42(7):951.
2. Binh MBN, et al. MDM2 and CDK4 immunostainings are useful adjuncts in diagnosing well-differentiated and dedifferentiated liposarcoma subtypes: a comparative analysis of 559 soft tissue neoplasms with genetic data. Am J Surg Pathol. 2005;29(10):1340–7.
3. Creytens D. A contemporary review of myxoid adipocytic tumors. In: Seminars in diagnostic pathology. WB Saunders, Philadelphia; 2019.
4. Deyrup AT, et al. Fibrosarcoma-like lipomatous neoplasm: a reappraisal of so-called spindle cell liposarcoma defining a unique lipomatous tumor unrelated to other liposarcomas. Am J Surg Pathol. 2013;37(9):1373–8.
5. Faa G, Sciot R. Soft tissue tumors occurring in the perinatal/infancy setting: 1st part. J Pediatr Neonatal Individ Med. 2018;7(1):e070114.
6. WHO Classification of Tumours Editorial Board. Soft tissue and bone tumors. Lyon: IARC Press; 2020.
7. Goldblum JR, Folpe AL, Weiss SW. Enzinger and Weiss's soft tissue tumors: expert consult. Philadelphia: Elsevier Health Sciences; 2020.
8. Hornick JL. Practical soft tissue pathology: a diagnostic approach. Pattern recognition series. 2nd ed. Philadelphia: Elsevier Health Sciences; 2017.
9. Lindberg MR, Lindberg MR, Chang A. Diagnostic pathology: soft tissue tumors. Philadelphia: Elsevier Health Sciences; 2015.
10. Mariño-Enriquez A, et al. Atypical spindle cell lipomatous tumor. Am J Surg Pathol. 2017;41(2):234–44.
11. Mccarthy AJ, Chetty R. Tumours composed of fat are no longer a simple diagnosis: an overview of fatty tumours with a spindle cell component. J Clin Pathol. 2018;71(6):483–92.
12. Schaefer I-M, Fletcher CDM. Recent advances in the diagnosis of soft tissue tumours. Pathology. 2018;50(1):37–48.
13. Schaefer I-M, et al. Histologic appearance after preoperative radiation therapy for soft tissue sarcoma: assessment of the European Organization for Research and Treatment of cancer–soft tissue and bone sarcoma group response score. Int J Radiat Oncol Biol Phys. 2017;98(2):375–83.
14. Wei S, et al. Soft tissue tumor immunohistochemistry update: illustrative examples of diagnostic pearls to avoid pitfalls. Arch Pathol Lab Med. 2017;141(8):1072–91.
15. Zaidi MY, et al. The impact of unplanned excisions of truncal/extremity soft tissue sarcomas: a multi-institutional propensity score analysis from the US sarcoma collaborative. J Surg Oncol. 2019;120:332.

Vascular Tumors

2

Raf Sciot, Clara Gerosa, Giuseppe Floris, Daniela Fanni, Maria Debiec-Rychter, and Gavino Faa

Introduction

Soft tissue vascular tumors represent a very high number of tumors, characterized by a wide clinical, morphologic and immunohistochemical spectrum. Because of major differences in their clinical behavior and, consequently, in treatment and prognosis, distinguishing vascular tumor entities represents an important challenge for surgical pathologists involved in the diagnosis of soft tissue tumors.

Various classifications exist and following subgroups may be identified:

A. Malformative vascular lesions
B. Classical vasoformative tumors
C. Reactive vascular lesions
D. Vascular tumors with hobnail endothelium
E. Spindled vascular tumors
F. Epithelioid vascular tumors

Various immunohistochemical markers are available. The most interesting and useful ones are as follows:

- *CD31*: stains virtually all endothelia/vascular lesions in a membranous pattern. A pitfall is the labeling of macrophages by this marker.

R. Sciot · G. Floris
Department of Pathology, KU Leuven, UZ Gasthuisberg, Leuven, Belgium

C. Gerosa · D. Fanni (✉) · G. Faa
Divisione di Anatomia Patologica, Dipartimento di Scienze Mediche e Sanità Pubblica, Università degli Studi di Cagliari, Azienda Ospedaliero-Universitaria di Cagliari, Cagliari, Italy

M. Debiec-Rychter
Department of Human Genetics, KU Leuven, UZ Gasthuisberg, Leuven, Belgium

© Springer Nature Switzerland AG 2020
R. Sciot et al. (eds.), *Adipocytic, Vascular and Skeletal Muscle Tumors*, Current Clinical Pathology, https://doi.org/10.1007/978-3-030-37460-0_2

- *ERG*: stains the nuclei of virtually all endothelial/vascular lesions. Can also be expressed in some epithelioid sarcomas, about half of prostate carcinomas, rare Ewing sarcomas, chloromas, cartilage tumors, normal lymphocytes.
- *Podoplanin (D2-40):* labels lymphatic endothelium, Kaposi sarcoma, +/− 50% of angiosarcomas. Can be expressed in many non-mesenchymal tumors.
- *Alpha-smooth muscle actin (alpha-SMA):* stains perivascular pericytes/ muscle cells.
- *Human herpesvirus 8 (HHV8):* highly sensitive and specific marker for Kaposi sarcoma, showing a nuclear and granular expression.
- *C-MYC*: overexpressed and amplified in secondary angiosarcoma (post-radiation or post-lymphedema) and also in some primary angiosarcomas.

In addition, numerous other markers are available with variable specificity and sensitivity. *CD34* is an endothelial marker but it also stains so many other mesenchymal lesions and is often lost in angiosarcoma. *GLUT-1* is positive in infantile hemangioma and some rapidly involuting congenital hemangiomas. *WT1* is often negative in malformative lesions and positive in tumors.

The purpose of this chapter is to evaluate the morphological, imunohistochemical, cytogenetic, and clinical characteristics of vascular tumors, with the aim of giving surgical pathologists a pattern-based approach, enabling to interpret this complex group of soft tissue neoplasms easier and more reproducible.

Malformative Vascular Lesions

Definition Vascular malformations are aggregates of vessels devoid of a normal organization that may be superficial or deep-seated. The distinction from real vascular neoplasms is on pure morphology often very difficult.

Age at Presentation Superficial vascular malformations are often diagnosed at birth, often being diagnosed as hemangiomas.

Classification It is mainly based on the constituent vessel type and size (i.e., capillary, lymphatic, venous, or arterial), mixed type vessels being frequent. They are frequently associated with clinical syndromes.

Syndromes
A. Rendu-Osler-Weber syndrome
B. Klippel-Trenaunay syndrome (capillary-venous-lymphatic malformations)
C. Parkes Weber syndrome (capillary-arteriovenous-lymphatic malformations)
D. PIKC3A-related overgrowth syndrome
E. Fibro-adipose vascular anomaly
F. PTEN hamartoma syndrome
G. Arteriovenous malformations (AVM) of brain

Classical Vasoformative Tumors

Capillary (Lobular) Hemangioma (Fig. 2.1)

Definition Lobular proliferation of dilated capillaries that may be superficial, deep, or intravenous. When superficial and polypoid, the term *pyogenic granuloma* is often used.

Age at Presentation Peaks between 10 and 30 years. Has a wide age range.

Gender No sex predilection.

Localization Head and neck > trunk > fingers > mucosal (gingival location is associated with pregnancy).

Clinical Presentation Rapid growth with evolution toward a fibrous papule.

Macroscopy Small red papule, pedunculated, or sessile; bleeding may occur. Often ulcerated.

Histology Lobules of capillaries separated by fibrous septa. Superficial capillaries dilated, deep capillaries tightly packed, with inconspicuous lumina (Fig. 2.2a). Non-atypical endothelium. Frequent mitoses. Neutrophils are often present. Superficial ulceration is frequently found. An epidermal collarette is typical for the classical pyogenic granuloma. Occasionally an intravascular growth is seen.

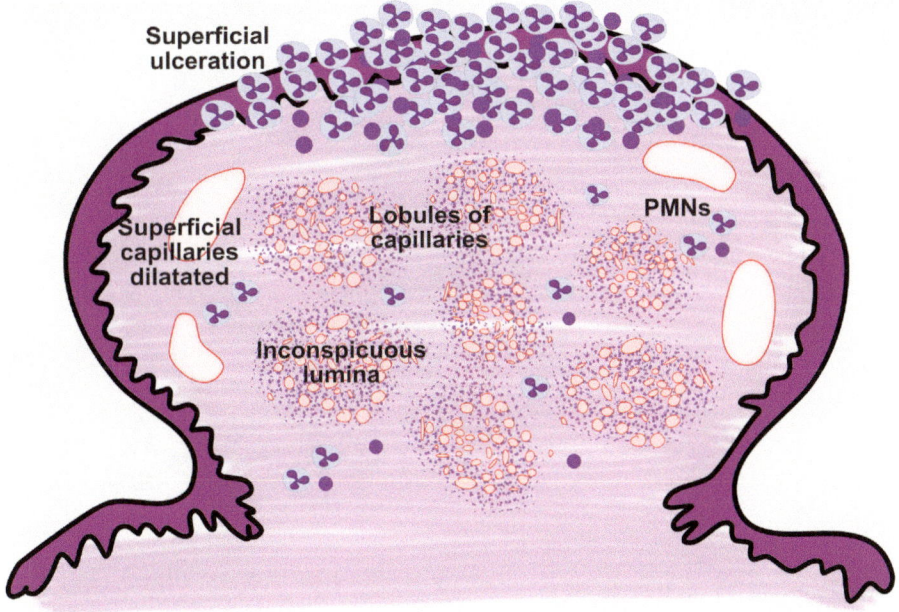

Fig. 2.1 Schematic representation of lobular capillary hemangioma

Fig. 2.2 Lobular capillary hemangioma in the hand of a 23-year-old female: HE-stained section, showing the lobular arrangement (**a**), immunohistochemistry for CD31 (**b**), and alpha-smooth muscle actin (**c**)

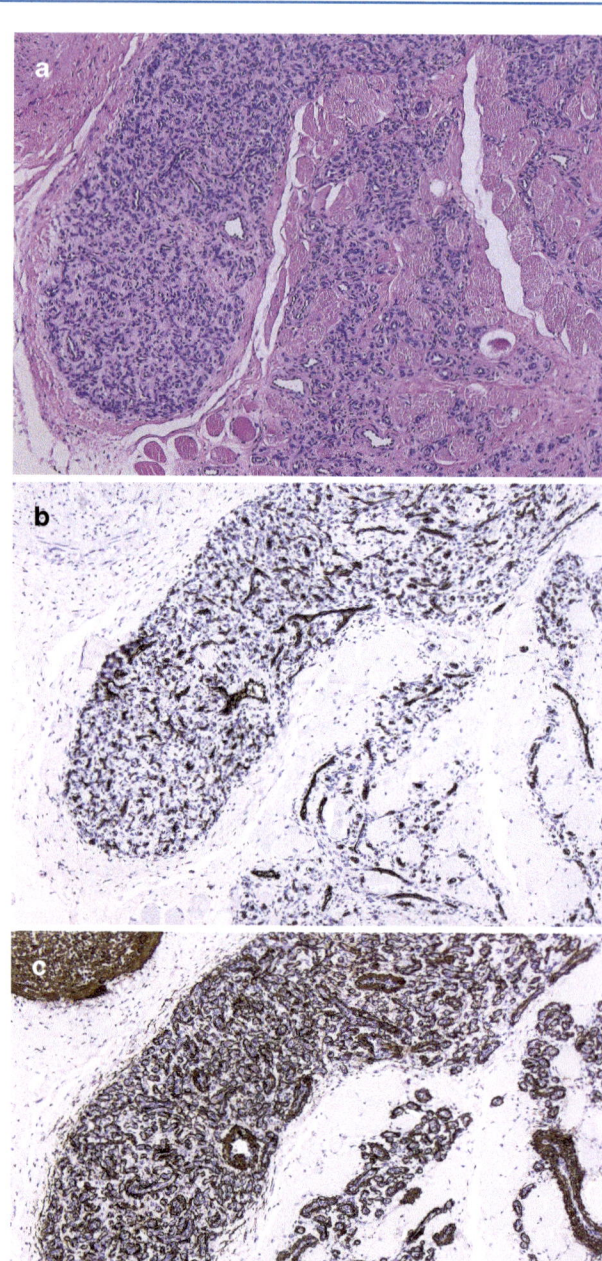

Immunohistochemistry GLUT1 is negative. All the other classical endothelial markers (CD31, CD34, ERG) are expressed (Fig. 2.2b). The vessels are delineated by an alpha-smooth muscle actin positive cuff (Fig. 2.2c).

Molecular Genetics No specific changes.

Prognosis Benign lesion.

Differential Diagnosis (DD) (1) *Juvenile capillary hemangioma* (JCH). Both share a lobular architecture and high mitotic rate. JCH is positive for GLUT-1. (2) *Nasopharyngeal angiofibroma:* this arises from the roof of the nasal cavity, whereas nasal capillary lobular hemangioma arises more from the septum. (1) *Cherry angioma*: it lacks the typical lobular architecture and occurs in adults.

Congenital Hemangioma

Definition A hemangioma that matures at birth, having undergone a proliferative phase in utero.

Age at Presentation It is evident at birth.

Gender Boys and girls are equally affected.

Localization Head & neck, trunk, limbs.

Clinical Presentation Two subgroups are described. (1) RICH: rapidly involuting congenital hemangioma, which regresses within +/− 1 yr and (2) NICH: non-involuting congenital hemangioma, which does not regress.

Macroscopy Superficial lesions appear as macules pink-bright red in color. Deep lesions present as bluish nodules.

Histology RICH shows the picture of a lobular capillary hemangioma (Fig. 2.3a, b), NICH contains dysplastic veins/arteries between the capillary lobules (Fig. 2.4a, b).

Immunohistochemistry RICH can show a weak/focal GLUT1 expression (Fig. 2.5a, b), NICH is GLUT1 negative (Fig. 2.5c, d).

Molecular Genetics Both can have *GNAQ* or *GNA11* mutations.

Prognosis Cfr. Clinical presentation.

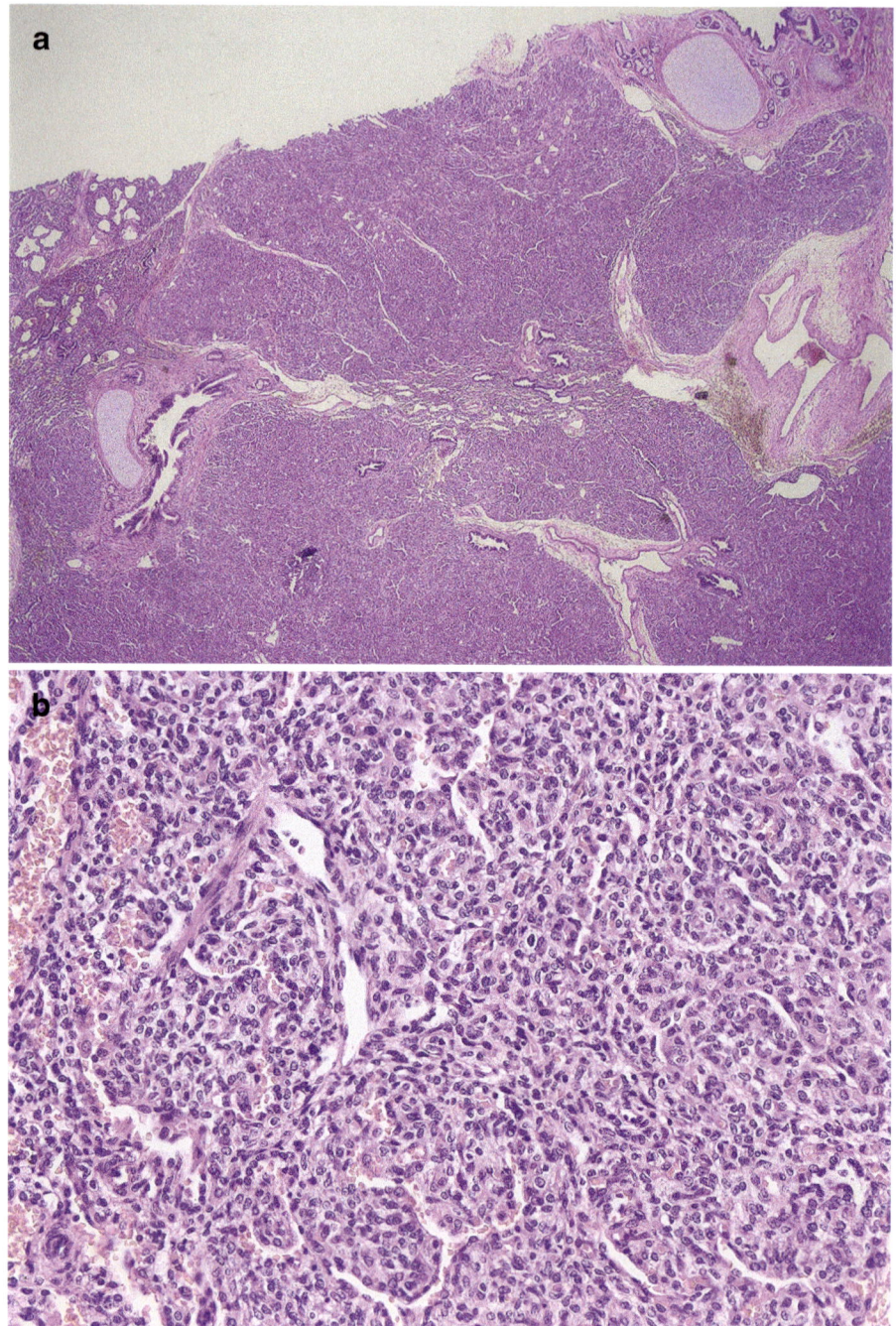

Fig. 2.3 Congenital hemangioma RICH in the lung of a female at birth: low-power (**a**) and high-power field (**b**) (HE-stained section), showing the tightly packed capillaries

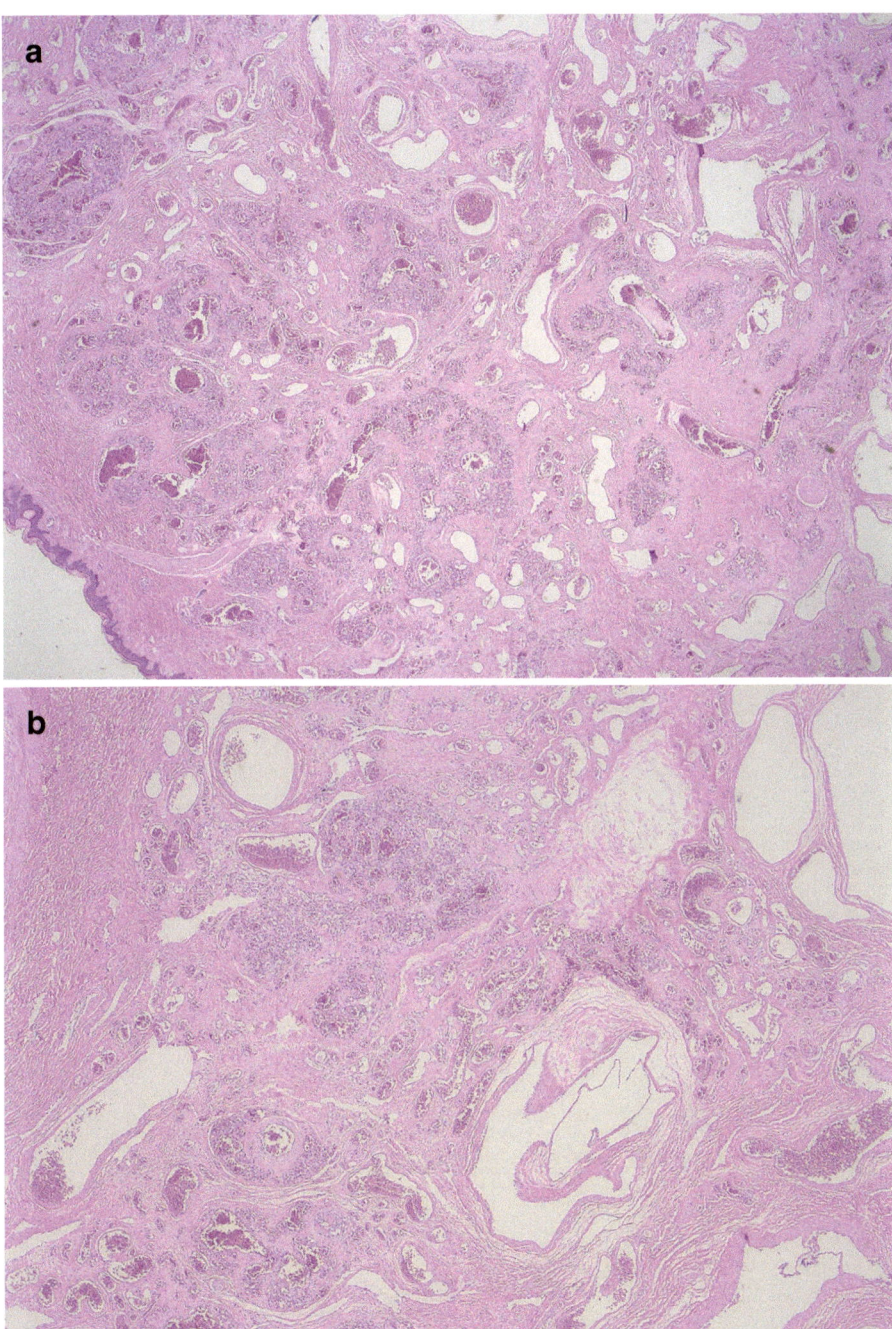

Fig. 2.4 Congenital hemangioma NICH at low-power (**a**) and high-power (**b**) field magnification in a 5-year-old boy, having this vascular lesion in his knee since birth and showing no improvement on taking Inderal (HE-stained section). Note the dysplastic larges vessels

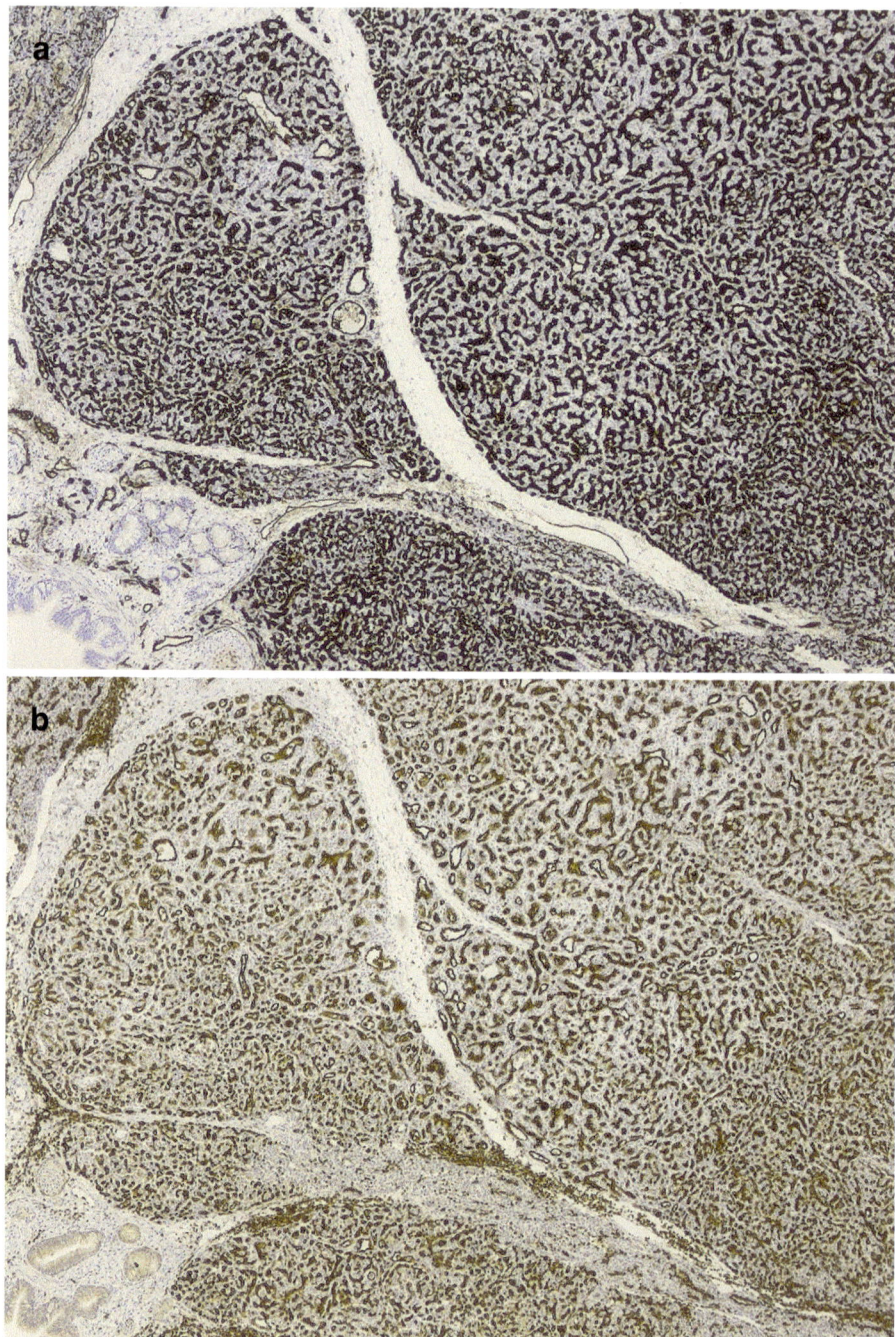

Fig. 2.5 Immunohistochemistry for CD31 (**a**) and GLUT1 (**b**) in congenital hemangioma RICH and for GLUT1 (only erythrocytes are stained) (**c**) and CD31 (**d**) in congenital hemangioma NICH

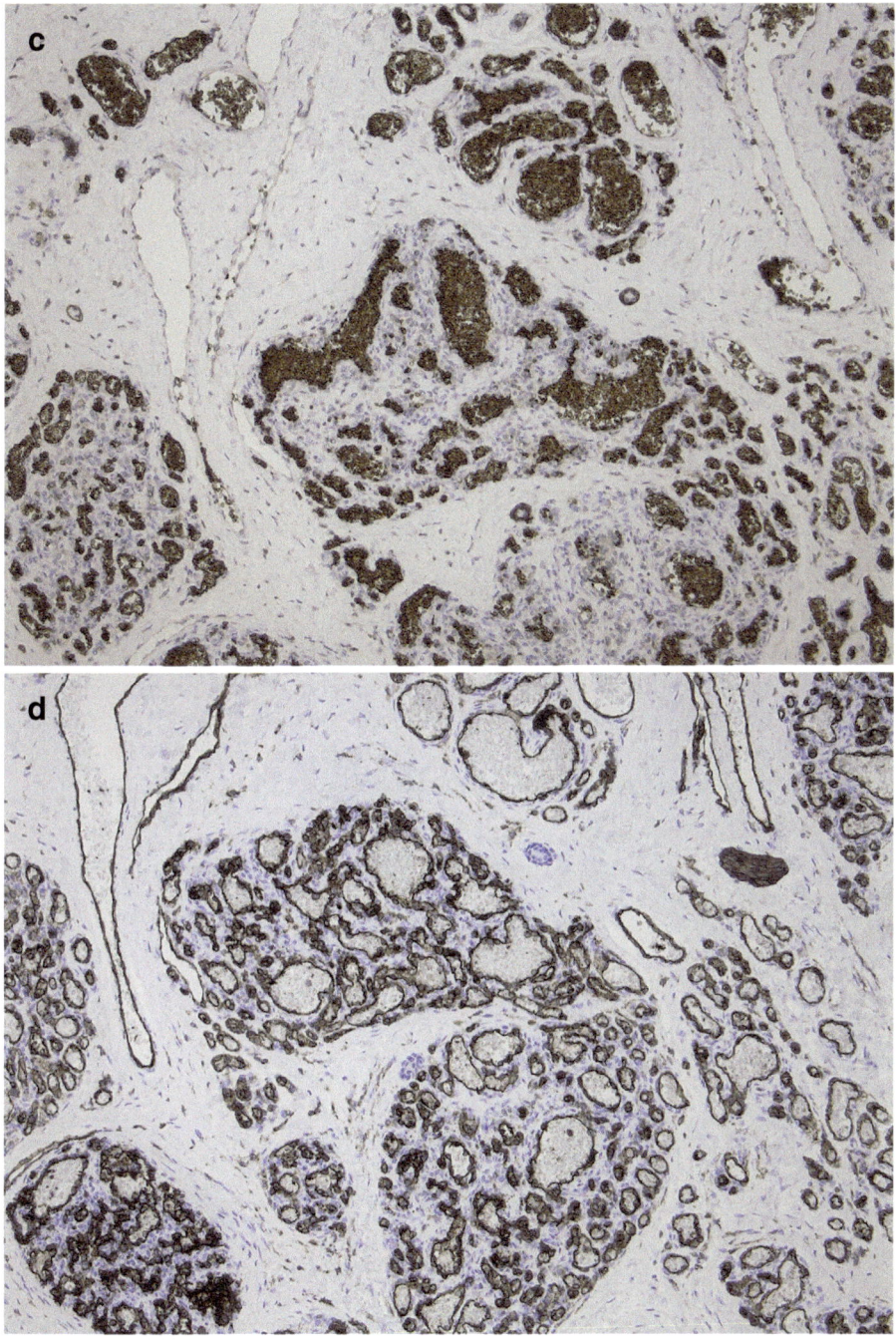

Fig. 2.5 (continued)

Infantile/Juvenile Hemangioma (Fig. 2.6)

Definition It is the most frequent hemangioma of infancy, affecting 4% of children.

Age at Presentation Often present in the first year of life. Preterm infants are more affected.

Gender Female predominance 3:1.

Localization Head and neck (50%), trunk, extremities.

Clinical Presentation Growth phase (6–12 months); involuting phase (1–12 years); end stage (normal skin).

Macroscopy At birth, superficial tumors appear as a pink macule that modifies into a bright-red macule during the growth phase. During the involuting phase, the color changes from red to pink, ending with a normal skin or a slightly discolored area. Deep intramuscular lesions appear as bluish nodules.

Microscopy Lobules of tightly packed capillaries appear mainly in the dermis, some nodules extending into the subcutaneous fat. Nodules show a solid pattern due to the poor canalization of capillaries and to plump endothelial cells. Mitoses are frequent. Pericytes are prominent. Inside the lobules, no interlobular stroma is observed. At the periphery of the lesion, well-canalized larger vessels are often found. Mast cells are sometimes abundant (Fig. 2.7a, b).

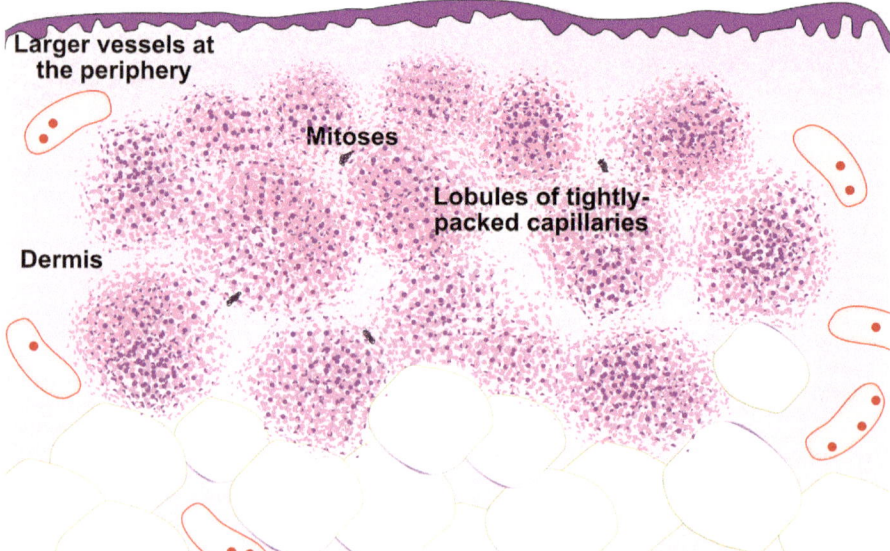

Fig. 2.6 Schematic representation of infantile (juvenile) hemangioma

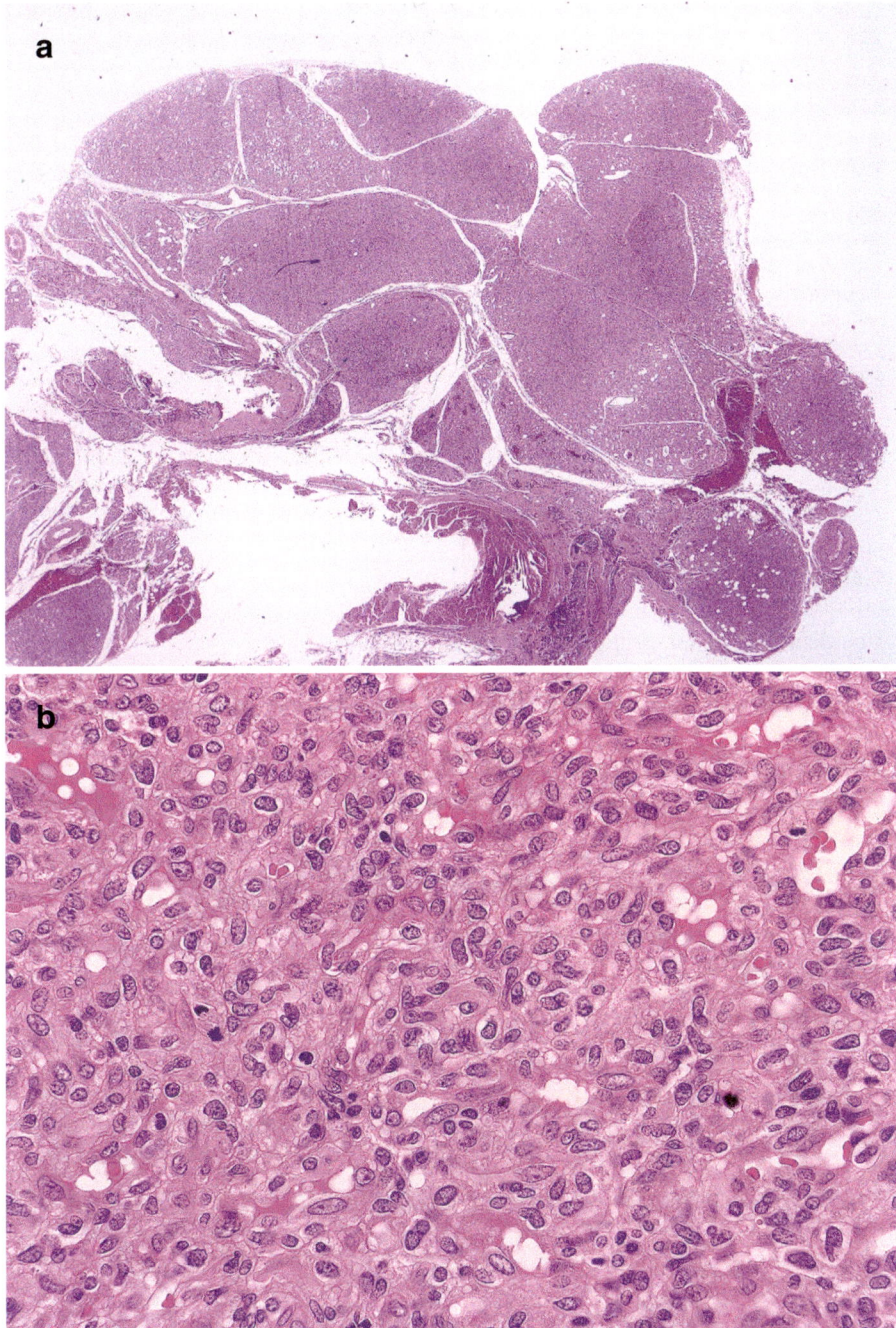

Fig. 2.7 Infantile (juvenile) hemangioma at low-power (**a**) and high-power field (**b**) (HE-stained section) in the neck of a 1-year-old girl. Mitoses are easily found in this dense lobular capillary proliferation

Immunohistochemistry Immunostaining for GLUT1 is strong and diffuse in endothelial cells. Alpha-SMA reactivity highlights the high number of pericytes.

Molecular Genetics No significant changes.

Differential Diagnosis (1) *Lobular capillary hemangioma:* capillary lobules are separated by dense fibrous septa; epidermal collarette is present; absence of GLUT1 on immunostaining is typical.

Prognosis Masterful neglect, propranolol can be effective.

Cherry (Senile) Hemangioma (Fig. 2.8)

Definition Most common skin vascular lesion of adults.

Age at Presentation From middle adulthood, increasing with age.

Gender No sex predilection.

Localization Trunk > upper extremities.

Clinical Presentation Small red papules that increase in number with age.

Microscopy Polypoid lesion within the superficial dermis consisting of dilated congested capillaries/venules, with thickened wall. No fibrous capsule. Thinning of

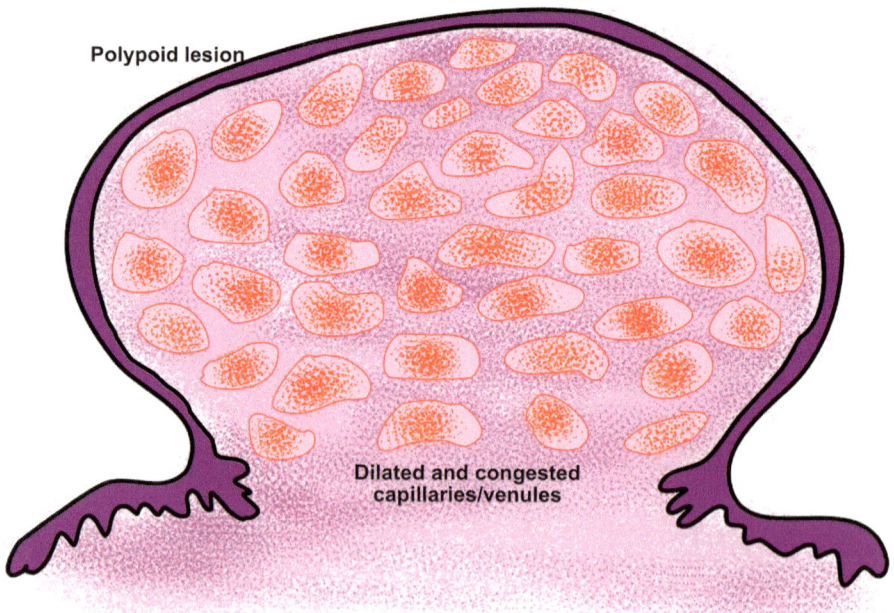

Fig. 2.8 Schematic representation of senile hemangioma

the overlying epidermis. Epidermal collarette often present. No lobular pattern. Rare mitoses (Fig. 2.9a, b).

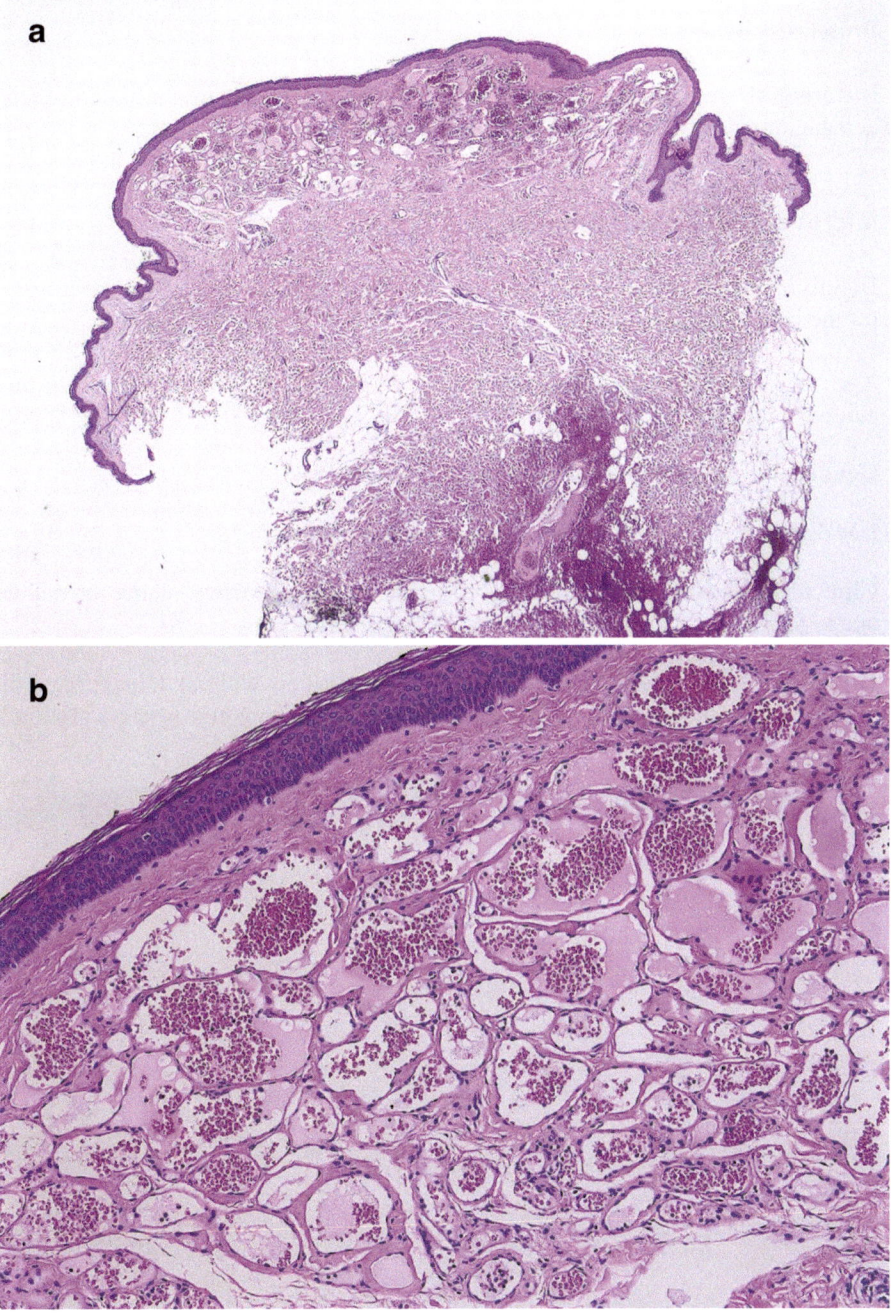

Fig. 2.9 Senile hemangioma at low-power (**a**) and high-power field (**b**) (HE-stained section) in the leg of an 80-year-old female. Note the superficial dilated vessels

Immunohistochemistry No particular changes.

Molecular Genetics *GNA14/GNAQ/GNA11* mutations have been described.

Prognosis Benign lesion.

Differential Diagnosis (1) *Lobular capillary hemangioma* in adulthood: cherry hemangioma lacks lobular architecture and mitoses are rare or absent.

Microvenular Hemangioma (Fig. 2.10)

Definition Rare benign cutaneous vascular tumor, characterized by a predilection for the limbs of young adults.

Age at Presentation Mean age: 39 years. Range: 1–70 years. Young adults > children > elderly people.

Gender No sex predilection.

Localization Extremities (limbs) > chest > back > abdomen.

Clinical Presentation Asymptomatic, stable or slow-growing, plaque or nodule, one to few centimeters in diameter, red to purple in color.

Histology It is a dermal poorly circumscribed lesion without lobulation. Thin venules, irregularly branched, compressed by the surrounding sclerotic reticular

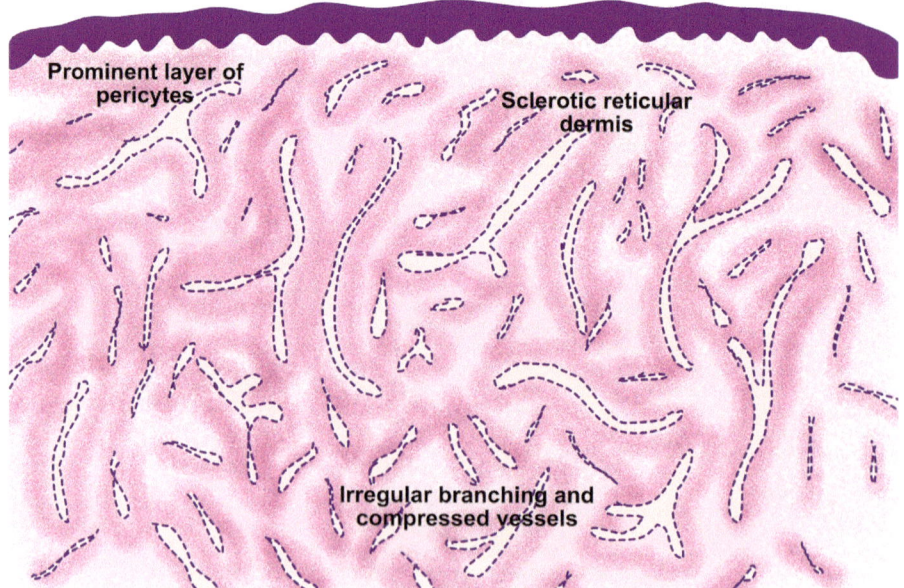

Fig. 2.10 Schematic representation of microvenular hemangioma

dermis. The thin compressed veins are encircled by a prominent layer of pericytes. Endothelium is plump. No atypia. No mitosis. The involvement of the arrector pili muscle is a typical feature (Fig. 2.11a, b).

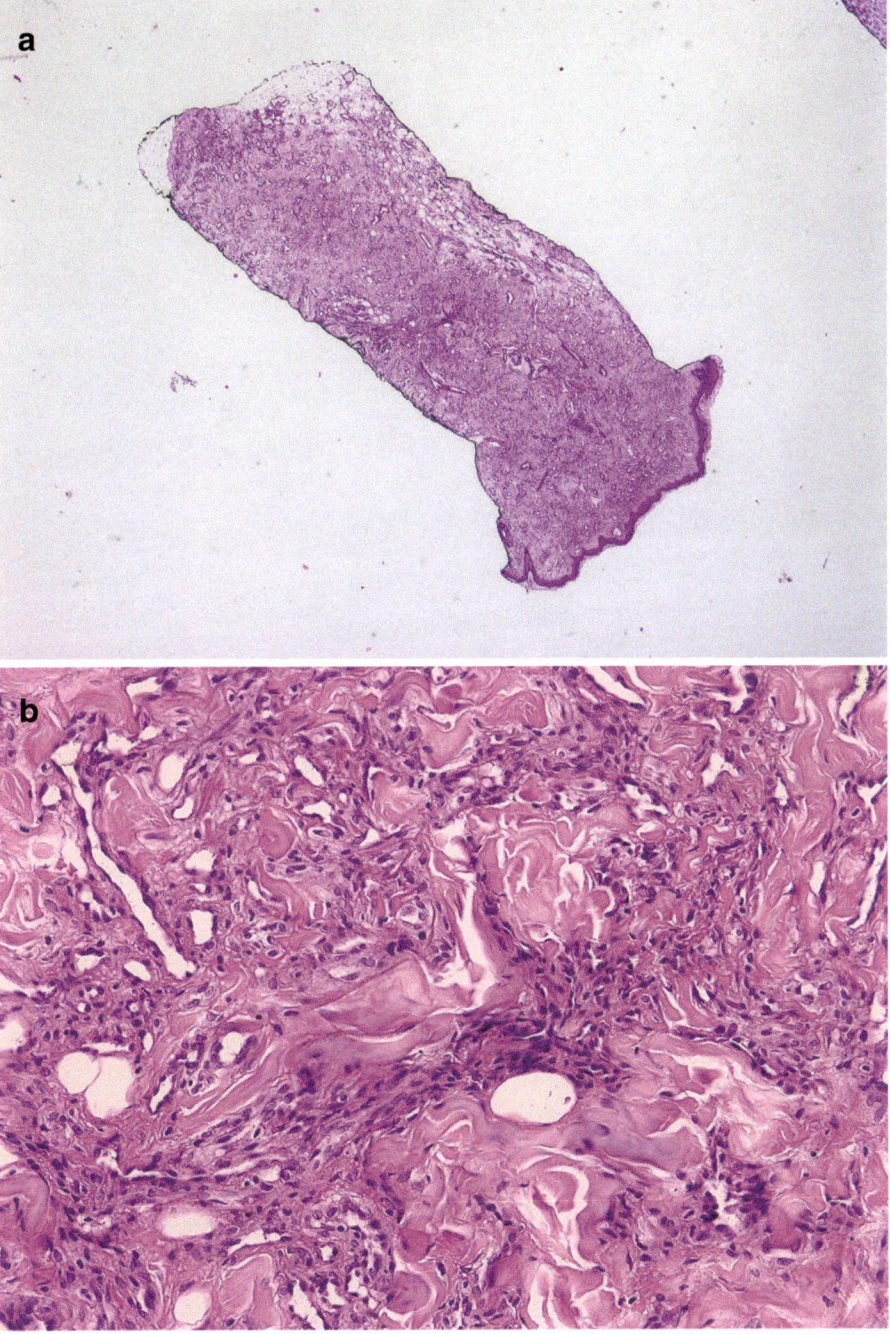

Fig. 2.11 Microvenular hemangioma at low- (**a**) and high-power field (**b**) (HE-stained section) in the upper arm of a 7-year-old boy. The vessels have a prominent perivascular cuff

Immunohistochemistry Strong alpha-SMA reactivity around each compressed vascular structure is a classical finding (Fig. 2.12a, b).

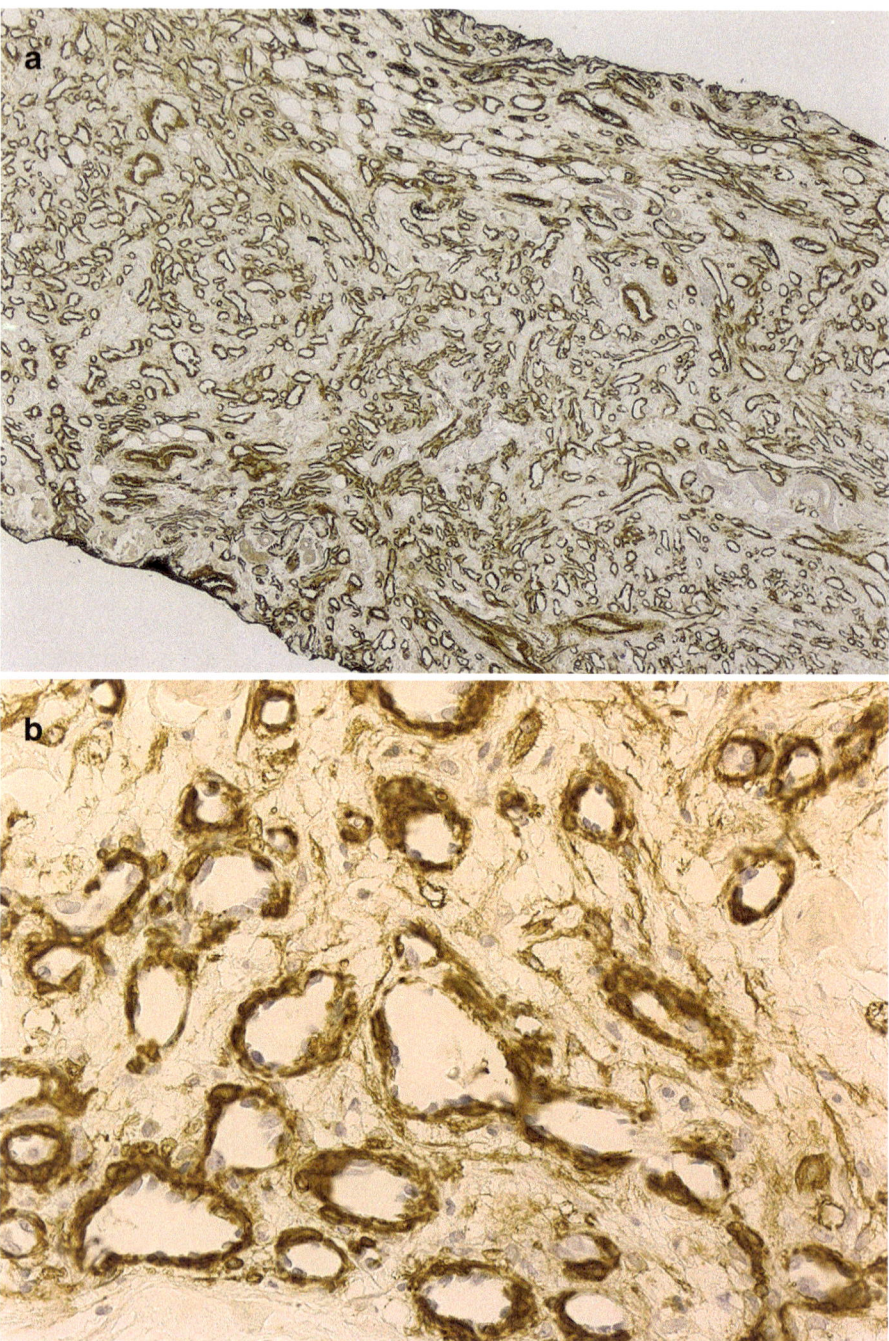

Fig. 2.12 Immunohistochemistry for SMA in microvenular hemangioma at low- (**a**) and high-power fields (**b**)

Molecular Genetics Not useful.

Prognosis Benign lesion.

Differential Diagnosis (1) *Kaposi sarcoma* (patch stage): erythrocyte extravasation; hemosiderin deposits; lymphoplasmocytic infiltrate; a spindle cell component; immunoreactivity for HHV8; lack of alpha-SMA-reactive pericytes.

Caveat At low power, in cases in which the involved dermis is particularly dense and sclerotic, compressed venules may not be easily identified, leading to a diagnosis of "normal skin." A careful, high-power-field examination may be mandatory in order to reach a correct diagnosis.

Cavernous Hemangioma (Fig. 2.13)

Definition Benign vascular tumor consisting of enlarged, thin-walled blood vessels.

Age at Presentation Infancy > childhood > adulthood.

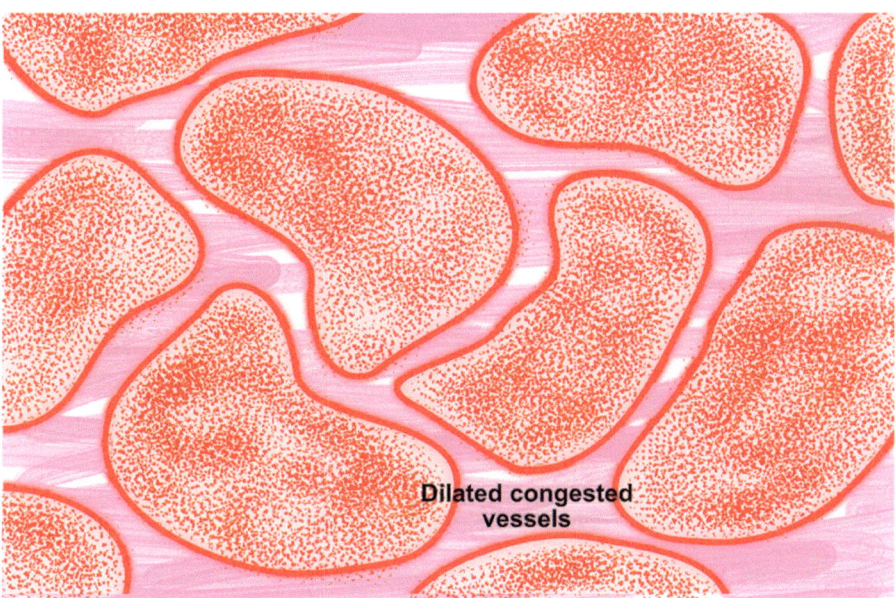

Dilated congested vessels

Fig. 2.13 Schematic representation of cavernous hemangioma

Localization The scalp, face, and neck are the most common sites, but these tumors have been found in organs and bone.

Clinical Presentation It presents as a soft, bluish mass. Large cavernous hemangiomas may be associated with consumptive coagulopathy, characterized by low-serum fibrinogen levels and high D-dimer levels, due to activation of coagulation inside the lesion.

Macroscopy A bluish soft area with a spongy consistency.

Histology Circumscribed proliferation of dilated thin-walled congested vessels (Fig. 2.14).

Variants (A) Sinusoidal hemangioma (Fig. 2.15). It has a preferential localization in the subcutaneous tissue of the mammary gland. The histological picture is

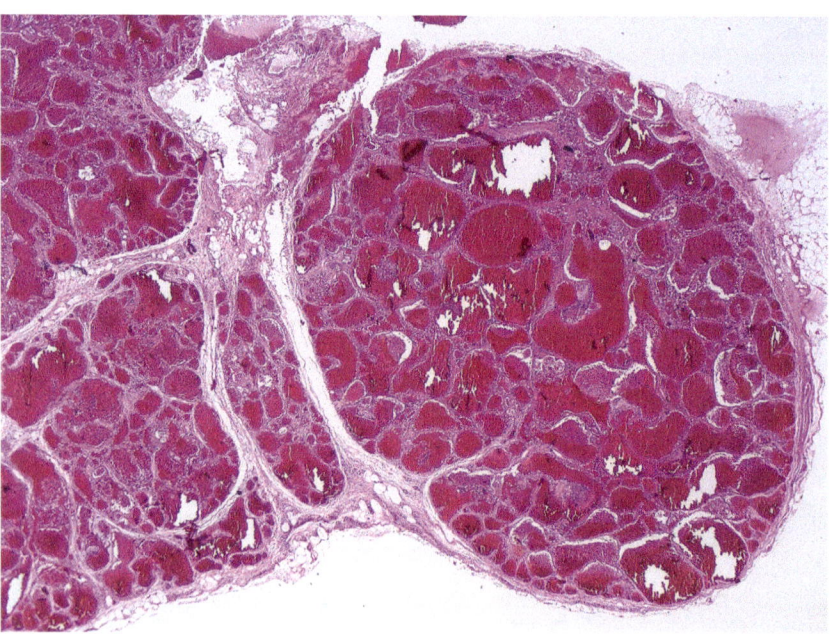

Fig. 2.14 Cavernous hemangioma (HE-stained section)

characterized by widely dilated vascular channels (sinusoids) and by back-to-back congested thin vessels with thrombi. Foamy macrophages and cholesterol clefts are often present (Fig. 2.16a, b).

Immunohistochemistry No particular patterns.

Molecular Genetics No recurrent changes.

Prognosis Benign lesion. Treatment includes observation, irradiation, sclerosing solutions, and laser surgery and excisional surgery.

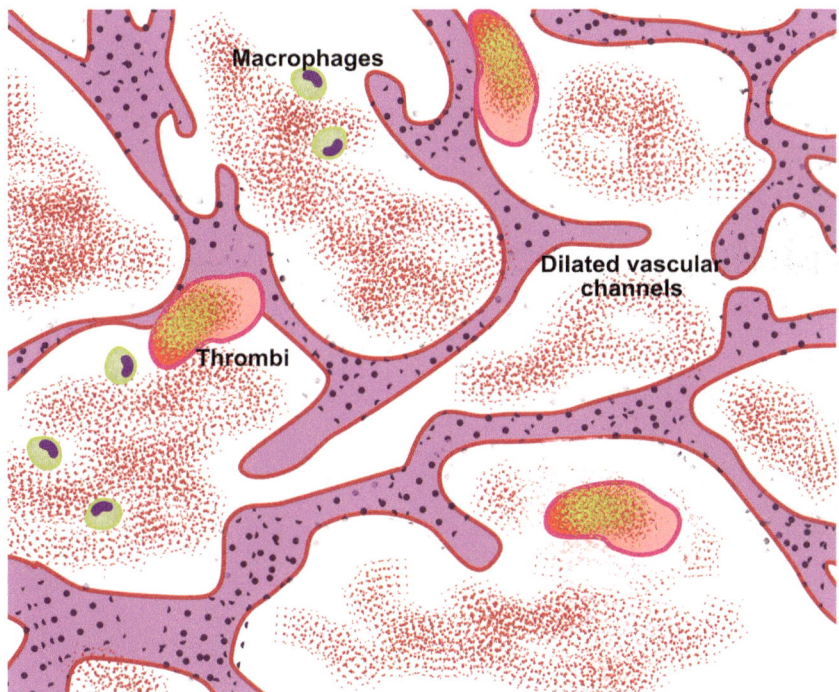

Fig. 2.15   Schematic representation of sinusoidal hemangioma

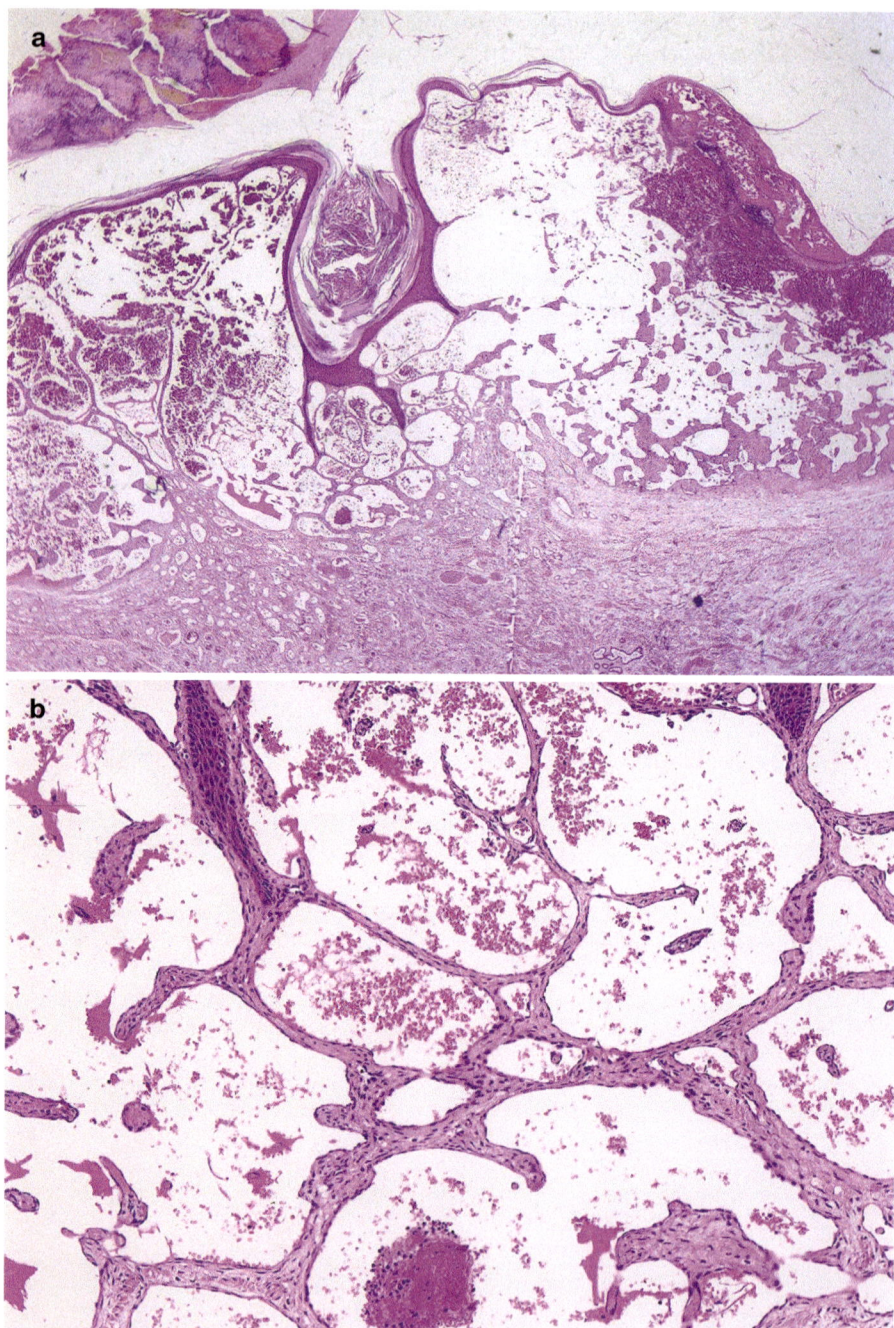

Fig. 2.16 1.6 cm nodular sinusoidal hemangioma on the knee of a 59-year-old male at low- (**a**) and high-power fields (**b**) (HE-stained section)

Arteriovenous Hemangioma (Fig. 2.17)

Definition Also known as *cirsoid aneurism*, it is considered a venous hemangioma in which some vessels undergo arterialization, with a preferential location in the face.

Age at Presentation > 40 years (adulthood).

Gender No sex predilection.

Localization Lips > perioral region > nose > eyelids.

Clinical Course Small, dome-shaped, dermal red-blue lesion, mainly arising in the face.

Microscopy Well defined but unencapsulated. Thin vein-like vessels; thick fibromuscular artery-like vessels, devoid of elastic lamina; few capillaries. Frequent intravascular thrombi. Papillary endothelial hyperplasia and dystrophic calcifications may be present (Fig. 2.18a, b).

Immunohistochemistry No diagnostic role.

Molecular Genetics *MAP2K1* mutations have been described.

Prognosis Benign lesion. Surgery is curative.

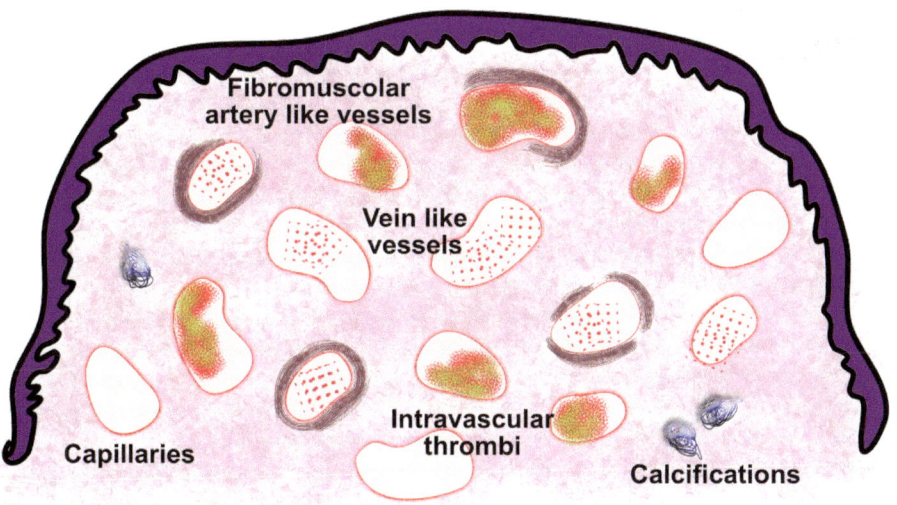

Fig. 2.17 Schematic representation of arteriovenous hemangioma

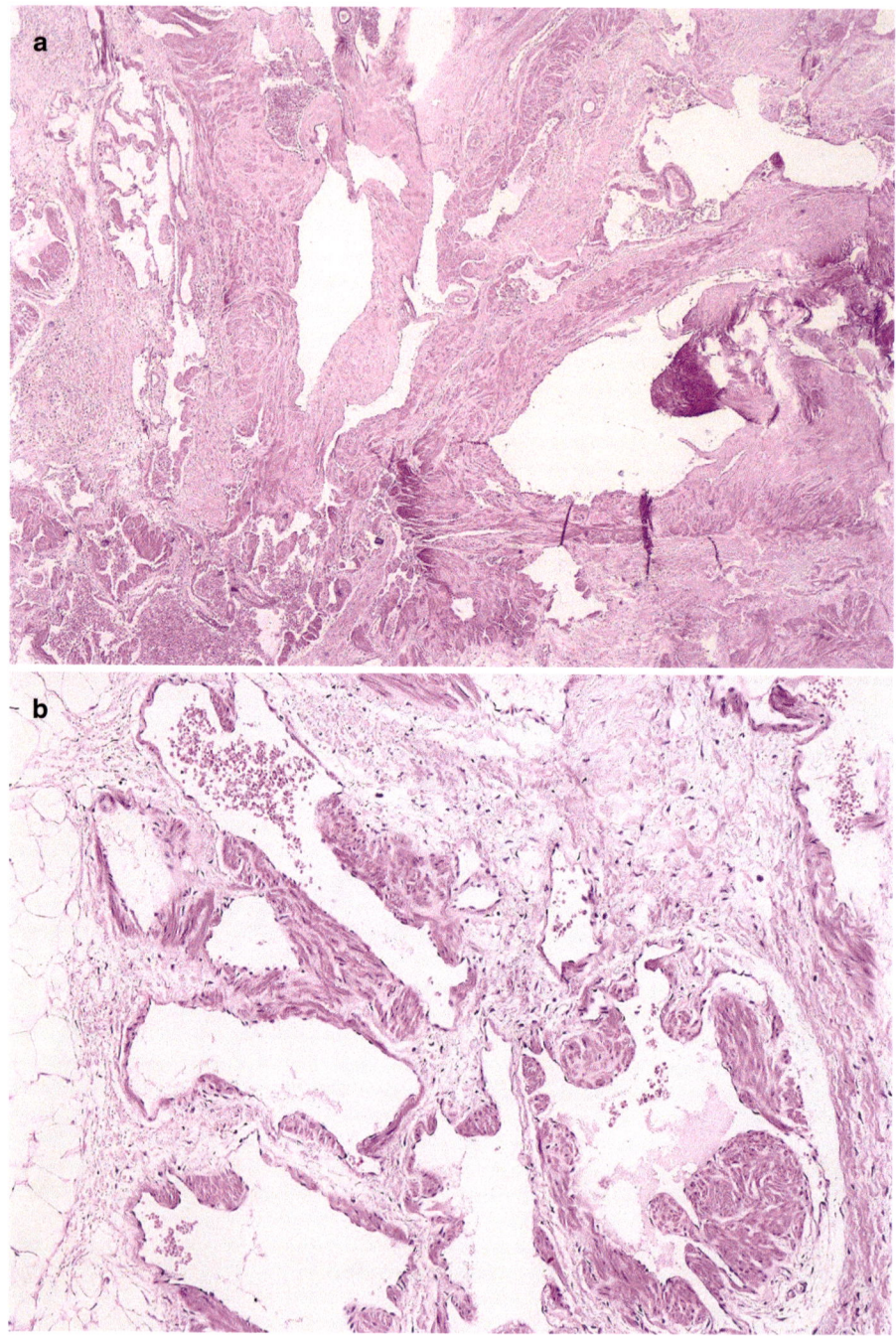

Fig. 2.18 Arteriovenous hemangioma in the upper leg of a 15-year-old male at low- (**a**) and high-power fields (**b**) (HE-stained section). Note the variable thickness of the vessel walls

Differential Diagnosis (1) *Arteriovenous malformation*: it frequently involves bone in the head and neck region; at histology, it is composed of large arteries, veins, and capillaries. Connection between arterious and venous channels is often seen.

Intramuscular Hemangioma (Fig. 2.19)

Definition Deep-seated hemangioma, generally considered a vascular malformation.

Age at Presentation <30 years. Rarely, it may present in adulthood.

Gender No sex predilection.

Localization Extremities > head and neck, always deep.

Clinical Presentation Painful deep lesion, with intermittent swelling.

Macroscopy Deep-seated mass.

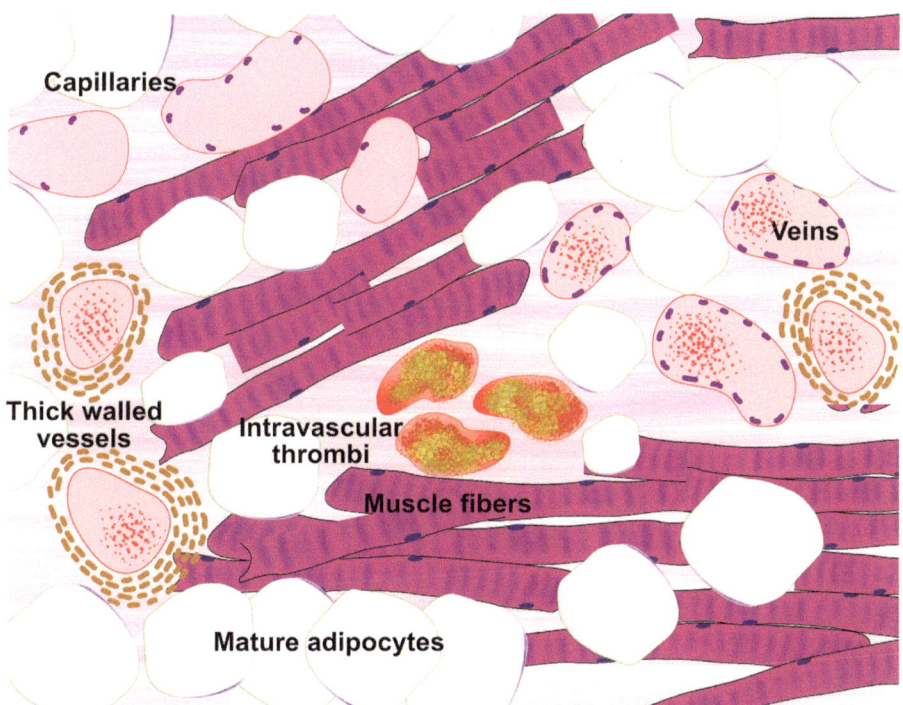

Fig. 2.19 Schematic representation of intramuscular hemangioma

Histology Mature adipocytes are almost always present, and they may be prominent. Mixed vessels, with veins predominating, often containing thrombi. Metaplastic ossification can be seen. Phleboliths are not uncommon (Fig. 2.20a, b).

Immunohistochemistry No distinctive immunohistochemical signature. Endothelial markers, including CD31 (Fig. 2.20c), are expressed.

Molecular Genetics No specific changes.

Prognosis Due to incomplete excision, recurrence rate is >60%. In asymptomatic patients, a wait-and-see approach is suggested. When necessary, sclerotherapy is preferred.

Angiomatosis

Definition Vascular malformation affecting subcutaneous tissue, muscle, and bone.

Age at Presentation Infancy or childhood.

Gender No sex predilection.

Localization Lowe extremities > trunk.

Clinical Course Progressive swelling, pain, discoloration of the affected area.

Macroscopy Affects a large segment of the body in a contiguous fashion, either by vertical extension to involve multiple tissue planes or by crossing muscle compartments to involve multiple muscles.

Histology Proliferation of thin veins, capillaries in clusters, and thick veins with fibrointimal hyperplasia. Mature adipocytes, fibrous septa, and nerve bundles are also observed.

Variants (A) The juvenile hemangioma-like variant is entirely formed by lobules of capillaries.

Molecular Genetics *PTEN/PIK3CA* mutations can be present.

Prognosis Complete surgical excision is rarely obtained, due to the extension of the lesion.

Differential Diagnosis *Juvenile hemangioma* may enter in differential diagnosis when the capillary proliferation predominates. The extension and depth of the lesion favor the diagnosis of angiomatosis.

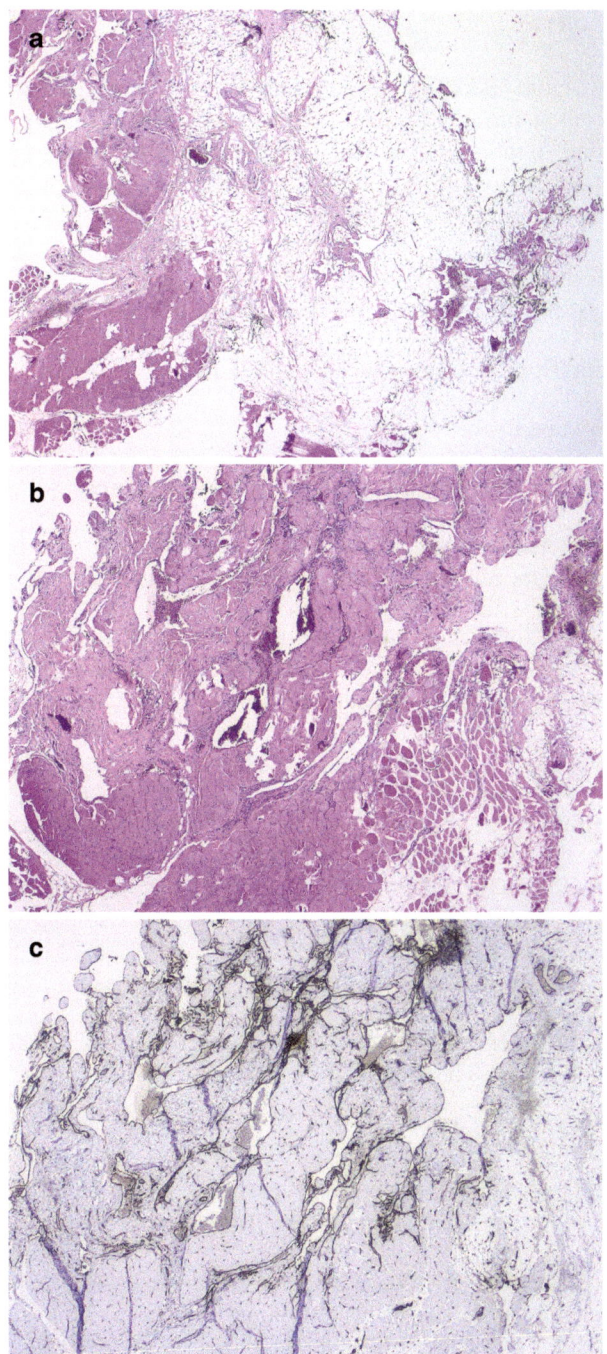

Fig. 2.20 Paravertebral intramuscular hemangioma in a 26-year-old male at low- (**a**) and high-power fields (**b**) (HE-stained section) and immunohistochemistry for CD31 (**c**). The fat component is prominent (**a**)

Lymphangioma

Definition Vascular lesion indistinguishable from a lymphatic malformation that usually presents at birth. Two main subtypes have been identified: a superficial microcystic one (lymphangioma circumscriptum) and a deeper macrocystic one (cavernous lymphangioma). Probably both represent a phenotypic spectrum of the same malformation.

Lymphangioma Circumscriptum
Definition It is the superficial microcystic subtype of lymphangioma.

Age at Presentation At birth or in early childhood.

Gender No sex predilection.

Localization Proximal extremities > limb girdles > scrotum.

Clinical Presentation Multiple superficial translucent vesicles, covering a skin area of one to several centimeter, that increase in number over time.

Macroscopy Multiple, small, clear, fluid-filled, clustered vesicles and papules that may resemble a gelatinous mass. Vesicles are different in color, translucent, pink, or red, due to hemorrhages from adjacent capillaries. Hyperkeratosis of the overlying skin, with verrucous appearance, is a frequent finding.

Histology Dilated thin-walled vascular spaces, localized beneath the epidermis, covered by a thin layer of endothelial cells. A chronic inflammatory infiltrate is often seen in the surrounding dermis. Verrucous lesions are characterized by epidermal hyperplasia (acanthosis) encircling the dilated lymphatic vessels.

Cavernous Lymphangioma
Definition It is a deep macrocystic subtype of lymphangioma.

Age at Presentation First two years of life. May be detected in adulthood when cutaneous involvement is absent.

Gender No sex predilection.

Localization Head and neck (hygroma cystica colli) > trunk > extremities > intra-thoracic > intra-abdominal (mesenterial).

Clinical Presentation It depends on the localization. Intra-abdominal lymphangioma may present as acute peritonitis.

Macroscopy Numerous translucent vesicles, increasing in number over time. Rarely, the vesicles may be deep-seated, including intrathoracic, intra-abdominal, and peritoneal localizations.

Microscopy Multiple large lymphatic channels, irregular in shape. A smooth muscle component can occasionally be detectable in the cystic wall. Lymphatic channels appear intermingled with lobules of adipocytes and with lymphoid aggregates. Fibrous septa may be detected (Fig. 2.21a, b).

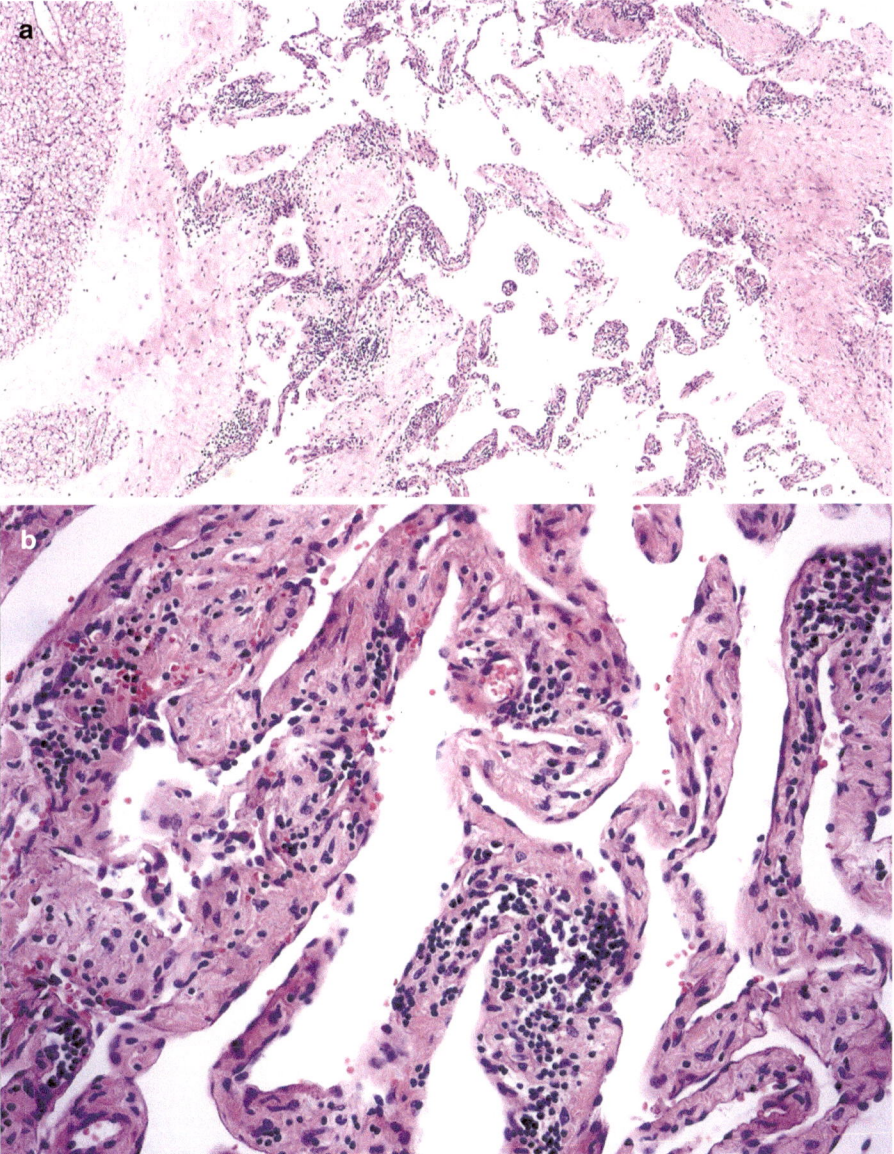

Fig. 2.21 Retroperitoneal cavernous lymphangioma in a 1-year-old boy at low- (**a**) and high-power fields (**b**) (HE-stained section). Lymfoid aggregates are easily seen

Variants Marked reactive changes, including myofibroblastic proliferation, fat necrosis, hemosiderin deposits, and granulation tissue, may characterize intra-abdominal lesions.

Immunohistochemistry Podoplanin expression is seen.

Molecular Genetics *PIKC3A* mutations have been reported.

Prognosis It depends on the superficial or deep location. Surgical excision is curative. Failure to excise the deep lymphatic lesions results in recurrences.

Differential Diagnosis (1) *Multilocular peritoneal inclusion cysts (benign multicystic mesothelioma)*: cysts are characterized by epithelioid cells, with occasional papillary structures. No muscle cell is present in the cystic wall. Keratins are highly expressed by the epithelium covering the cystic spaces.

Benign Lymphangioendothelioma

Definition Also known as acquired progressive lymphangioma, it is a rare benign lesion that, due to some atypical features, may be misinterpreted as Kaposi sarcoma or angiosarcoma.

Age at Presentation It usually presents during adolescence to young adulthood, but congenital cases have been described.

Gender Similar incidence in females and males.

Localization Skin, all sites, including lips.

Clinical Presentation Erythematous, slowly growing patch or plaque, few centimeters in size. The lesion is generally solitary, but multiple lesions have been occasionally reported.

Macroscopy It presents as a large, red-to-brown patch or plaque.

Microscopy Proliferation of anastomotic or retiform thin-walled vessels with a single layer of endothelial cells, dissecting the dermal collagen. Dermal structures are preserved but dissected and separated by anastomosing channels irregular in shape, giving rise to a pseudo-Kaposi or pseudo-angiosarcoma pattern. The majority of vascular channels are empty. The endothelium is thin, bland.

Immunohistochemistry D2-40 reactivity is observed in the endothelial cells.

Molecular Genetics No diagnostic change.

Prognosis Complete excision is curative. Recurrence is rare due to incomplete excision.

Differential Diagnosis (1) *Angiosarcoma*. The presence of a high mitotic index, of marked cytologic atypia, and of endothelial prominence and multi-layering are in favor of a malignant vascular tumor. (2) *Kaposi sarcoma*. It typically presents with multiple lesions, mainly on the lower extremities. A lymphoid and plasma cell infiltrate are often present. Immunostaining for HHV8 confirms the diagnosis of Kaposi sarcoma. (3) *Hobnail hemangioma*. A prominent hobnail endothelium associated with massive deposits of Perls-positive hemosiderin granules characterizes the picture of this lesion. (4) *Postradiation atypical vascular lesions*. The presence of radiotherapy in the clinical story is fundamental for this differential diagnosis.

Lymphangiomatosis

Definition A vascular malformation composed of lymphatic vessels, affecting large areas of the body, extending from the subcutaneous tissue to underlying muscles and bones. It may be systemic or localized.

Age at Presentation Infancy and childhood. The lesions may be present at birth.

Gender No sex predilection.

Localization Lower extremities and trunk in the localized form. In the systemic form, skin, soft tissues, gastrointestinal tract, mediastinum, retroperitoneum, bones, spleen, lungs, and pleura may be involved.

Clinical Course Progressive swelling and pain of the affected districts are the typical presenting symptoms.

Macroscopy Swelling of the affected zones.

Microscopy Multiple thin anastomosing empty cystic channels, dissecting the collagen bundles. The picture is similar to that of cavernous or cystic lymphangioma (Fig. 2.22).

Littoral Cell Angioma (LCA)

Definition Rare vascular tumor of the spleen arising from the cells that line the sinuses of the red pulp (littoral cells).

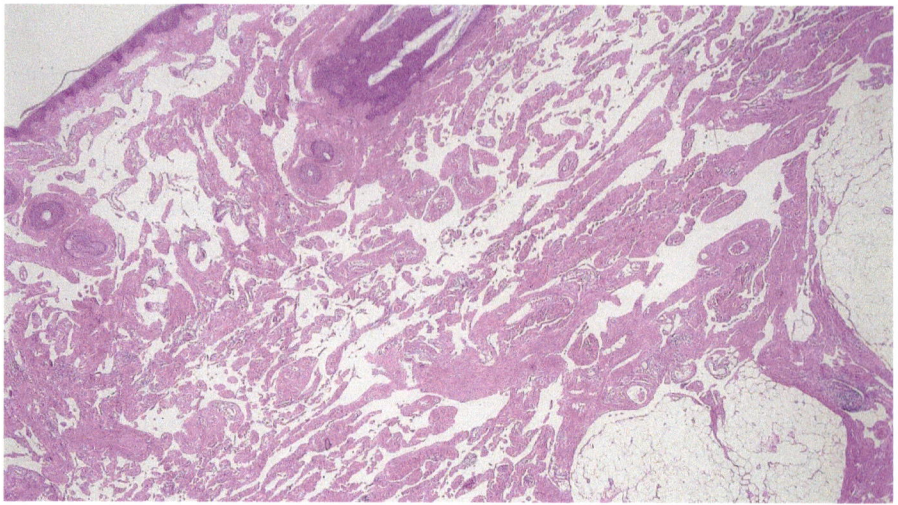

Fig. 2.22 Lymphangiomatosis from a boggy swelling of a whole right leg in a 14-year-old male (HE-stained section), showing the diffuse infiltrating character

Age at Presentation Young people.

Gender No sex predilection.

Localization Spleen.

Clinical Course The tumor may be asymptomatic for many years. Frequently, it is diagnosed incidentally. Splenic rupture may be the clinical presentation of LCA.

Macroscopy Often multiple spongy nodules.

Histology Unencapsulated nodular lesion, with pushing margins. Anastomosing small vascular channels and cystic spaces containing red blood cells. Vascular spaces are lined by tall plump endothelial cells. No atypia is detected. Papillary projections may be present (Fig. 2.23a, b).

Immunohistochemistry Littoral tumor cells are immunoreactive for CD31 and CD163. Unlike normal littoral cells, tumor cells of LCA are negative for CD8.

Molecular Genetics No specific change.

Prognosis Originally thought to be benign, recently LCA has been described as having some malignant potential. A close clinical follow-up is recommended.

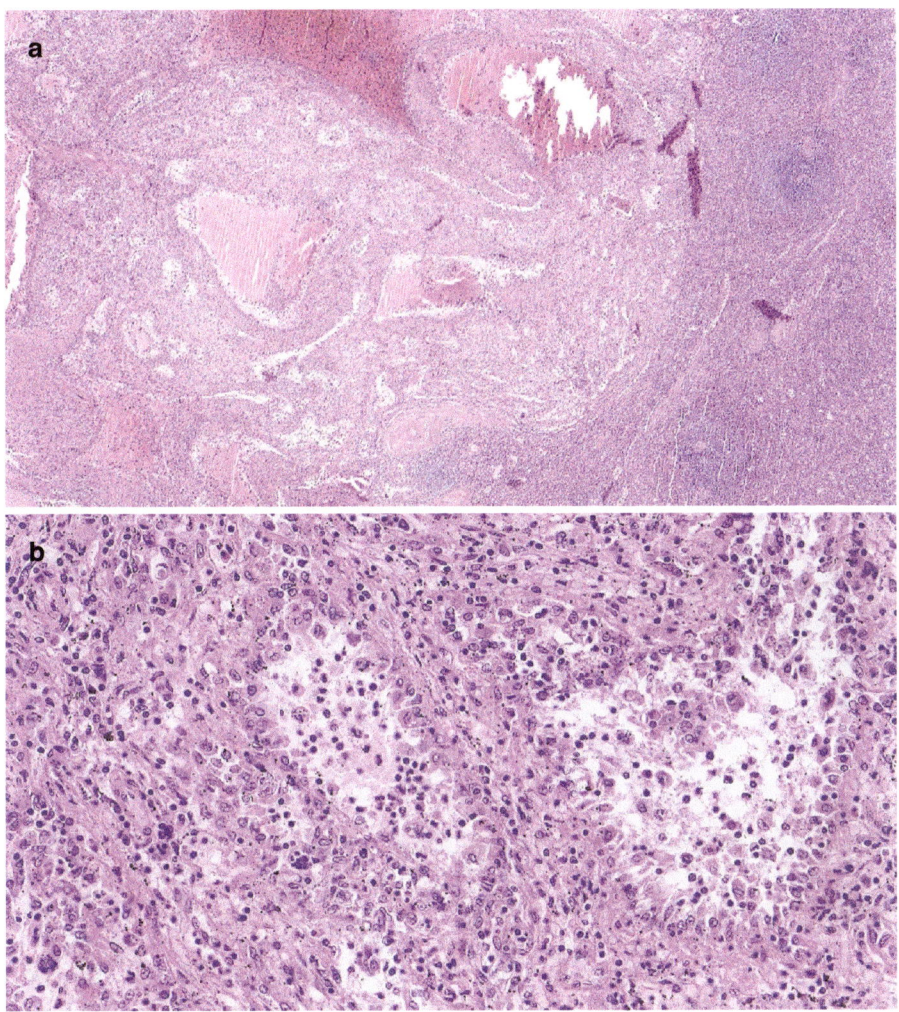

Fig. 2.23 Littoral cell angioma from a nodule in the spleen of a 38-year-old female at low- (**a**) and high-power fields (**b**) (HE-stained section), highlighting the plump delineating endothelial cells

Angiosarcoma (Fig. 2.24)

Definition   Rare malignant tumor characterized by blood vascular and/or lymphatic differentiation. According to the localization and the clinical setting, they may be subdivided into primary cutaneous angiosarcoma (the majority), angiosarcoma of deep soft tissue/bone and viscera, and post-radiotherapy/lymphedema angiosarcomas.

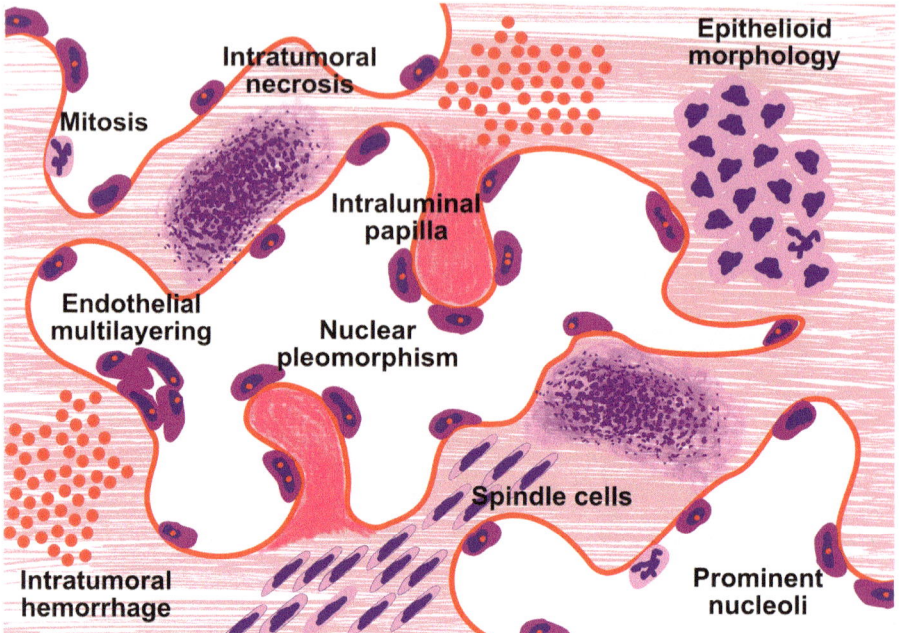

Fig. 2.24 Schematic representation of angiosarcoma

1. Soft Tissue/Visceral/Bone Angiosarcoma

Age at Presentation Children are rarely affected. Peaks in the seventh decade.

Gender No sex predilection.

Localization Retroperitoneum and extremities in adults. Visceral localization is rare, including liver, adrenal glands, gut, and thyroid. In children, mediastinum is the preferential site.

Clinical Course Sometimes soft tissue angiosarcoma can develop in the site of a previous hemangioma or vascular malformation, or after radiotherapy. Most lesions are sporadic and not associated with any previous lesion.

Macroscopy Enlarging painful mass, often associated with intratumoral hemorrhages or with hemorrhagic ascites or hemothorax according to the site of origin.

Histology Three main architectural patterns may be encountered: (i) *vasoformative*, characterized by thin walled vessels, irregular in shape, infiltrating the surrounding soft tissues, giving rise to the typical dissecting growth pattern. Cytology may be bland, or, more typically, neoplastic vessels are lined by atypical endothelial cells with dark enlarged prominent nuclei, with focal multilayering. Intraluminal papillary projection, lined by atypical protruding cells, may be seen; (ii) *solid* in which irregular infiltrating tumor vessels are characterized by a thin lumen and surrounded by a spindle cell to epithelioid component, with high mitotic index; in viscera and especially bone, tumors are often very epithelioid*;* (iii) *mixed,* with both components alternating in different fields. In low-grade cases, atypia of endothelial tumor cells may be very discrete, and diagnosis is based on the diffuse infiltrative growth pattern into the surrounding fat tissue. Mitoses are found both in vasoformative zones and more frequently in solid areas. Intratumoral hemorrhages are frequent, sometimes obscuring the neoplastic vascular structures, leading to diagnostic difficulties. In these cases, the diagnostic clue may be found at the periphery of the tumor mass. Intratumoral necrotic foci are frequently detected.

Immunohistochemistry CD31, ERG, and Fli1 reactivity are the typical markers of angiosarcoma. D2-40 is expressed in half of angiosarcomas. Keratin can be expressed in epithelioid types. Alpha-SMA positive cuffing is usually lacking.

Differential Diagnosis
A. *Benign vascular tumors*: the finding of a dissecting growth pattern, infiltrative margins, multilayering of atypical endothelial cells, and marked and diffuse cytological atypia of endothelial cells, associated with a high mitotic rate and intratumoral necrotic foci, favor the diagnosis of malignancy. The simple finding of a high mitotic index is not sufficient for a diagnosis of malignancy, which is also being found in some benign vascular tumors, particularly in children.
B. *Carcinoma*: The combination of an epithelioid phenotype and keratin expression may erroneously lead to the diagnosis of (metastatic) carcinoma. CD31 and ERG are mandatory in this context.

Molecular Pathology No consistent diagnostic changes.

Prognosis It is poor, particularly in tumor originating from the retroperitoneum in old patients.

2. Cutaneous Angiosarcoma.

Age at Presentation Elderly subjects.

Gender Predominant in males.

Localization Head and neck, sun-damaged skin.

Clinical Course Presenting symptoms: violaceous macule > plaque > nodule. Lesions may be multiple. With small lesions surrounding a central larger nodule.

Macroscopy Reddish plaque or nodule, with infiltrative margins.

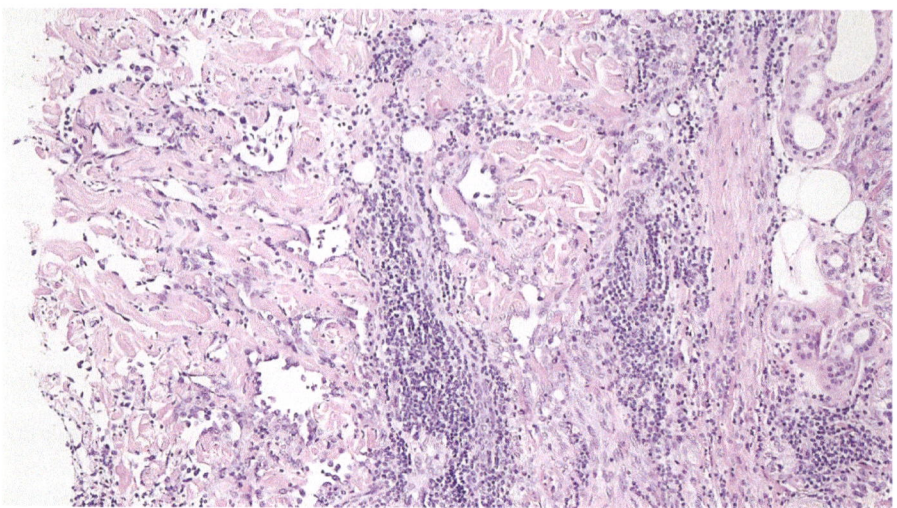

Fig. 2.25 Detail of a cutaneous angiosarcoma on the frontal skin of an 86-year-old male (HE-stained section). The dissecting pattern, atypical nuclei and inflammation are obvious

Histology The tumor mass is centered in the reticular dermis. The subcutaneous tissue is often infiltrated. An inflammatory component may be found, associated with hemosiderin granules and extravasated red blood cells. The tumor is often very dissecting and shows hyperchromatic nuclei and mitoses (Fig. 2.25).

Immunohistochemistry CD31, Fli1, and ERG are strongly and diffusely expressed by endothelial tumor cells. Alpha-SMA positive cuffing is usually lacking.

Molecular Genetics No consistent changes.

Prognosis Aggressive soft tissue tumor, with poor prognosis in the majority of cases. A diameter < 5 cm is considered a positive sign. The correlation between the histological grade and prognosis is debated.

3. *(Mammary) Angiosarcoma arising after radiation therapy will be discussed in a further chapter.*

Reactive Vascular Lesions

Papillary Endothelial Hyperplasia (PEH) (Fig. 2.26)

Definition Also known as hemangioma vegetans of Masson, PEH is a rare exuberant form of endothelial proliferation inside an organizing thrombus, often arising within a dilated vessel. Rare extravascular forms may occur. This reactive entity has the ability to mimic a variety of neoplastic diseases both benign and malignant.

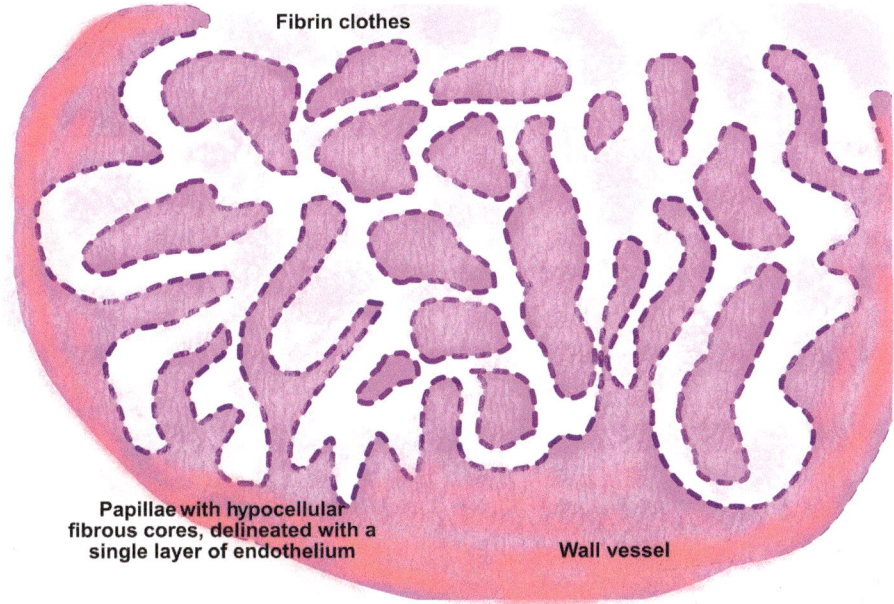

Fig. 2.26 Schematic representation of papillary endothelial hyperplasia

Age at Presentation Middle-aged people, usually in the fifth decade.

Gender Mild female preponderance, with a male/female ratio of 1: 1.3.

Localization Fingers>head and neck (orofacial region) > inflamed hemorrhoidal plexus.

Clinical Course Slow-growing mass.

Macroscopy At surgery, a nodule, reddish blue in color and firm in consistency, with small feeding blood vessels is observed.

Microscopy The histological picture is characterized by papillae with a hypocellular core, covered by flattened endothelial cells, with focally hyperchromatic prominent but not atypical nuclei. No significant atypia is found. Mitoses are rare or absent. Fibrin thrombi are often present. Granulation tissue is often found in the surroundings (Fig. 2.27a, b).

Immunohistochemistry No diagnostic role.

Molecular Genetics No reported changes.

Prognosis Surgical complete excision is curative.

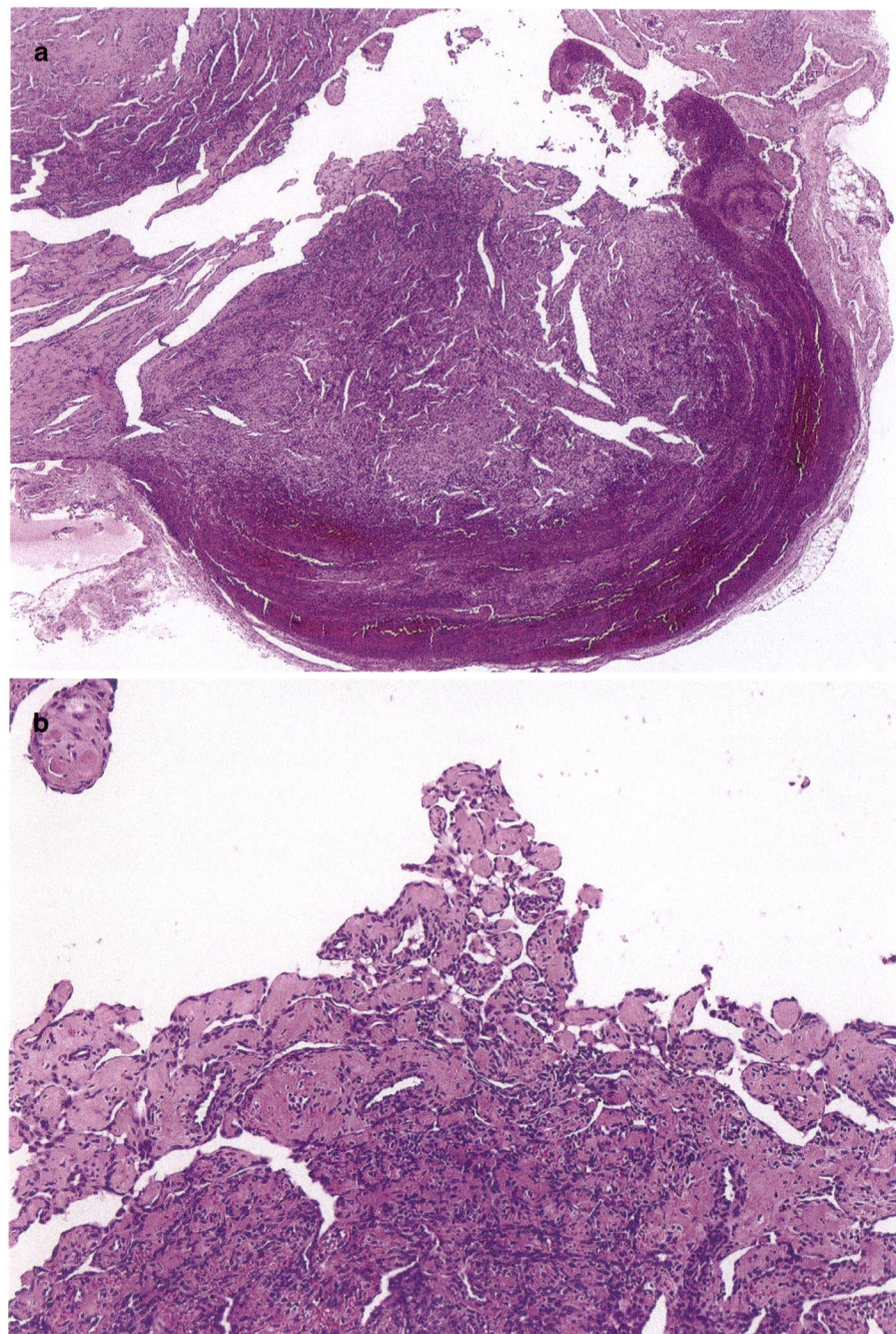

Fig. 2.27 Papillary endothelial hyperplasia from the finger of a 38-year-old female at low- (**a**) and high-power fields (**b**) (HE-stained section). Note the prominence of papillae

Differential Diagnosis The main DD is an angiosarcoma because of the papillary tufting, but PEH is devoid of atypia.

Bacillary Angiomatosis (Fig. 2.28)

Definition Reactive vascular proliferation induced by *Bartonella henselae* or *Bartonella quintana*, mainly occurring in HIV+ or HIV− immunodeficient subjects. More rarely, immunocompetent subjects may be affected.

Age at Presentation Adults.

Gender Females and males equally affected.

Localization Oral cavity > conjunctiva > lymph nodes > liver.

Clinical Course If untreated, red papules may disseminate.

Macroscopy Multiple red papules.

Histology Lobular capillary proliferation, localized in the subcutaneous tissue. Endothelial cells are plump, with mild to moderate atypia. Mitoses are frequent. Neutrophilic infiltrate is prominent in the myxoid stroma, associated with leukocytoclasia (nuclear dust). Violaceous clumps of bacteria may be detected. An epidermal collarette is often present (Fig. 2.29a–c).

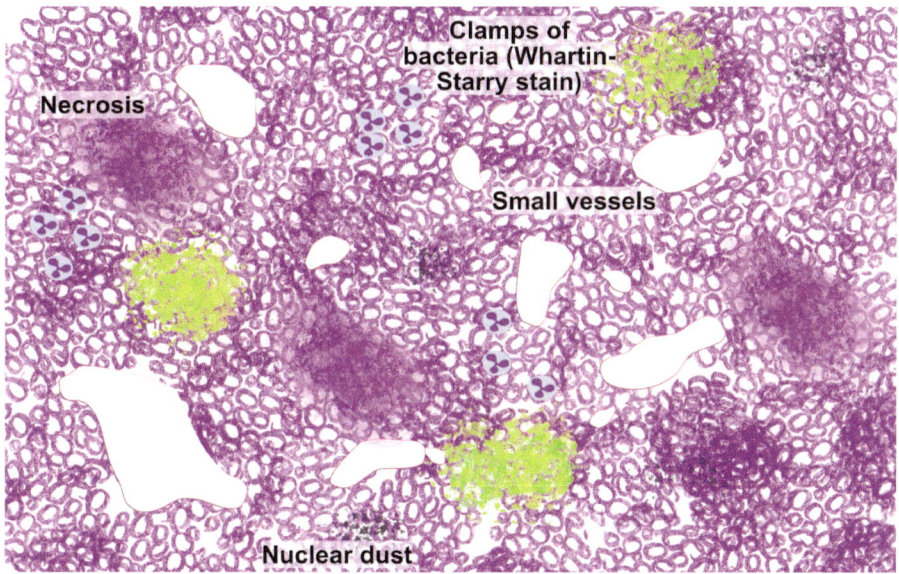

Fig. 2.28 Schematic representation of bacillary angiomatosis

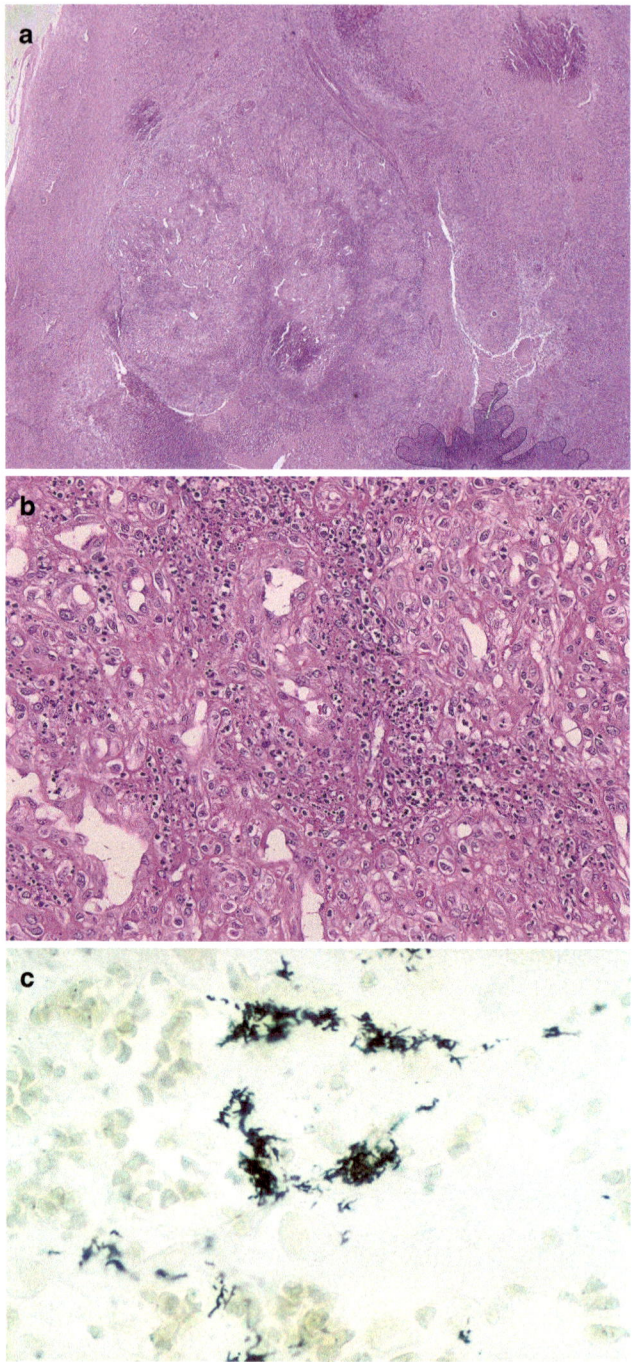

Fig. 2.29 Bacillary angiomatosis from the finger of a 38-year-old female at low- (a) and high-power fields (b) (HE-stained section) and with Whartin-Starry stain (c)

Immunohistochemistry No diagnostic role.

Molecular Genetics No specific changes.

Prognosis Appropriate antibiotic therapy with oral doxycycline is curative.

Differential Diagnosis (1) *Lobular capillary hemangioma:* The prominent neutrophilic infiltrate, nuclear dust, and clumps of bacteria are absent.

Reactive Angioendotheliomatosis (Fig. 2.30)

Definition Rare reactive cutaneous vascular proliferation, mainly occurring in adults affected by systemic diseases (lymphoma, chronic renal disease, liver failure, autoimmune liver disease).

Age at Presentation Adults. Rarely in infants.

Gender No sex predilection.

Localization Cutaneous lesions.

Clinical Course Dramatic presentation, with appearance of multiple patches and/ or papules (till 100), that may ulcerate and become necrotic.

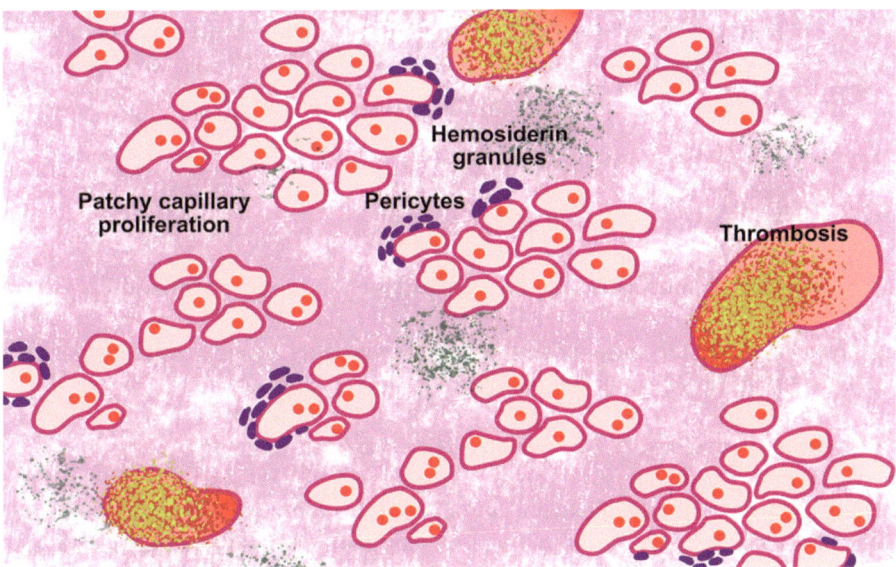

Fig. 2.30 Schematic representation of reactive angioendotheliomatosis

Macroscopy Multiple (hundreds) purpuric patches and plaques, few millimeter to several centimeter in diameter.

Histology At low power, the lesion is not well circumscribed. Proliferation of small capillaries surrounded by pericytes, arranged in small nests, scattered throughout dermal collagen fibers. Endothelial cells may show hobnail appearance and mild atypia. Mitoses are rare. Hemosiderin granules are present in the dermis. The histological pattern may change from one lesion to the next (Fig. 2.31a, b).

Immunohistochemistry Alpha-SMA, reveals a prominent pericytic component. Very rarely, occasional HHVV8 expression has been reported.

Molecular Genetics No reported changes.

Prognosis May change significantly from one patient to another. Some subjects respond to corticosteroid therapy, others are refractory. Treatment of underlying disease may reduce the lesions.

Differential Diagnosis (1) *Angiosarcoma*: the absence of multilayering, of severe cytological atypia, and of a high mitotic index, together with a strong reactivity for alpha-SMA, point against malignancy.

Glomeruloid Hemangioma (GH) (Fig. 2.32)

Definition It is a rare cutaneous, benign vascular tumor that appears to be characteristic for "polyneuropathy, organomegaly, endocrinopathy, monoclonal gammopathy, and skin changes syndrome" (POEMS). Rarely, GH may occur without an underlying POEMS syndrome.

Age at Presentation Young adults.

Gender No sex predilection.

Localization Trunk > proximal limbs. Rarely the face may be involved.

Clinical Course GH may present as small, multifocal vascular skin papules or as lesions with a cerebriform morphology.

Macroscopy Solitary or multiple blue-red papules or nodules.

Histology Dermal or subcutaneous localization of dilated vascular spaces with complex intravascular proliferations, resembling renal glomeruli. Intravascular proliferations are formed by small capillaries, with plump endothelium. PAS+ diastase-resistant hyaline globules are present (Fig. 2.33a, b).

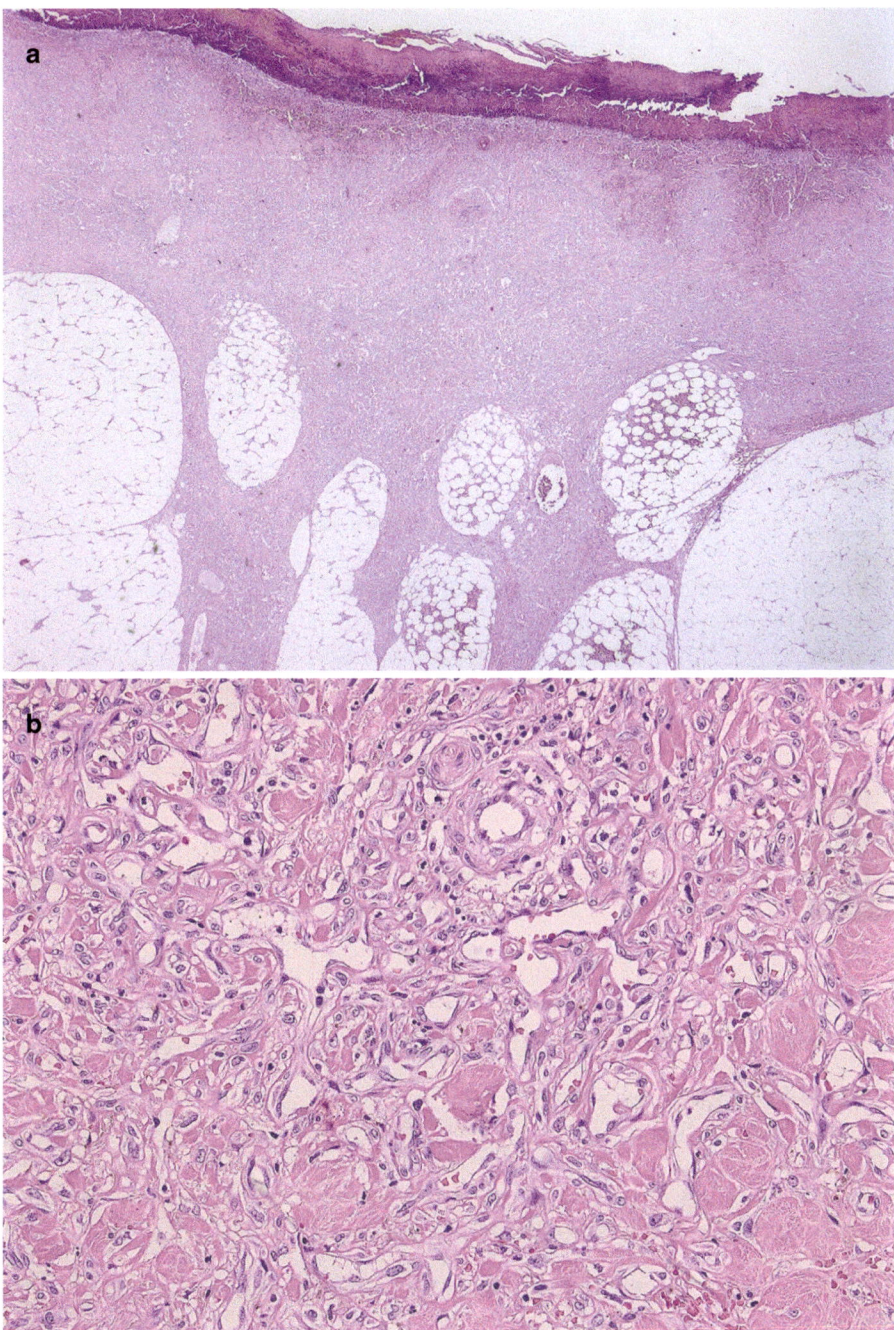

Fig. 2.31 Reactive angioendotheliomatosis from the kidney transplant of a 55-year-old male with elevated angiomatous lesion flank at low- (**a**) and high-power fields (**b**) (HE-stained section). The infiltrative character is obvious

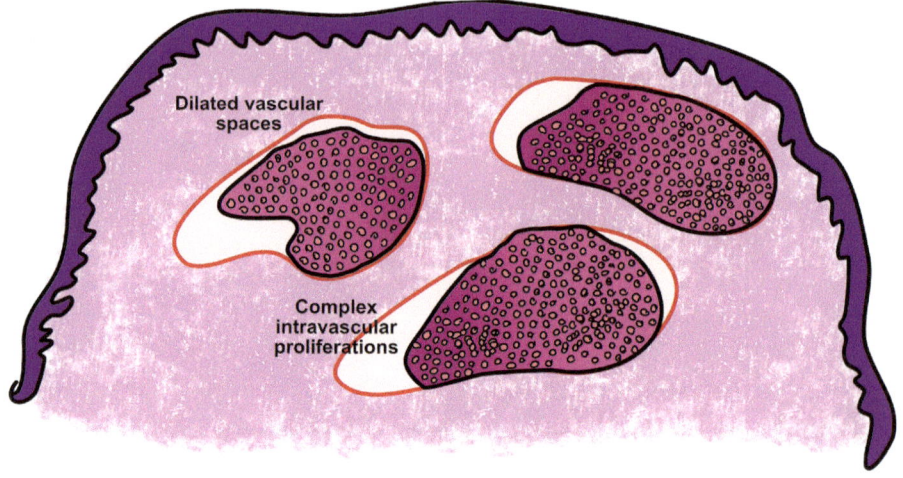

Fig. 2.32 Schematic representation of glomeruloid hemangioma

Immunohistochemistry No significant diagnostic role. Hyaline globules are reactive for immunoglobulin stains.

Molecular Genetics No specific change.

Prognosis Surgical resection is curative. Lesions may disappear after treatment of the underlying tumor (plasmacytoma, lymphoma).

Differential Diagnosis (1) *Papillary hemangioma*: it is a solitary lesion, presenting in healthy subjects and restricted to the head and neck region. Papillary structures show a fibrous core, covered by endothelial cells with intracytoplasmic abundant hyaline globules.

Vascular Tumors with Hobnail Endothelium

Hobnail Hemangioma (HH)

Definition Also known as targetoid hemosiderotic hemangioma, HH is a benign vascular cutaneous tumor characterized by large vascular channels covered by a hobnail endothelium, probably of lymphatic origin.

Age at Presentation Young adults. Wide range of age. Rarely congenital.

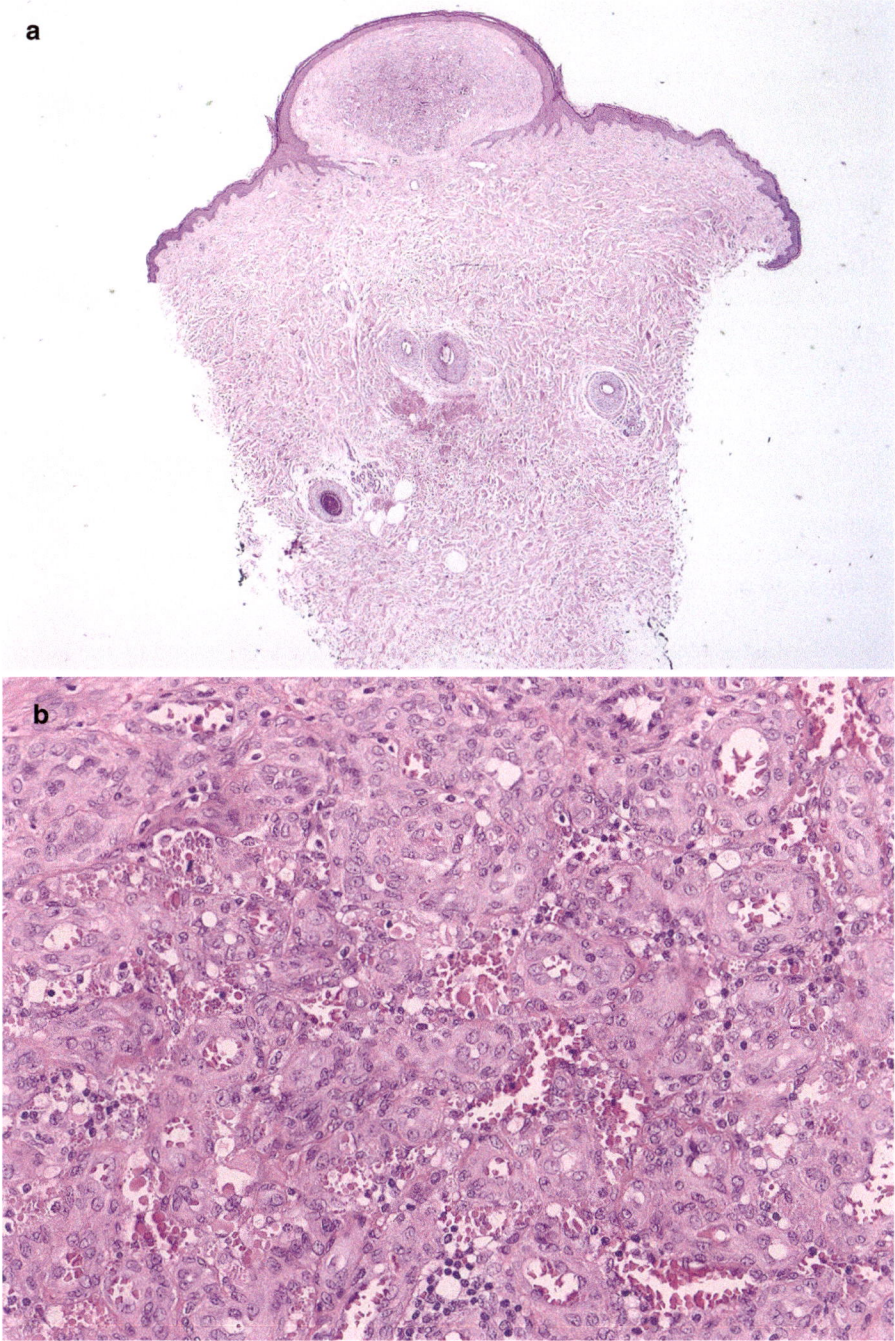

Fig. 2.33 Glomeruloid hemangioma at low- (**a**) and high-power fields (**b**) (HE-stained section) from a 31-year-old male, with multiple skin lesions. POEMS was diagnosed after the skin biopsy. At high power the glomeruloid clustes and hyaline globules are clearly present

Gender No sex predilection.

Localization Skin of extremities > trunk > head and neck.

Clinical Course HH presents with one (rarely multiple) papule or macule that may spontaneously involute and recur. In females, the lesion may change according to the menstrual cycle or in pregnancy.

Macroscopy The classical cutaneous lesion is a violaceous papule surrounded by a clear halo and by a peripheral ecchymotic zone that gives rise to a "target-like" appearance. HH may also present as a dusky red to brown papule or macule with a surrounding ecchymotic macular ring.

Histology A biphasic pattern is characteristic. (A) Dilated vascular channels in the upper dermis, covered by a hobnail endothelium bulging into the vascular lumen. Some channels contain erythrocytes, whereas others show a lymphatic-like appearance. Small intraluminal papillae may be present. (B) In the deep dermis, compressed vascular structures give rise to a dissection growth pattern. No extension is observed into the subcutaneous fat (Fig. 2.34a–c).

Immunohistochemistry CD31 and D2-40 are diffusely expressed by the hobnail epithelium. CD34 expression is focal or absent.

Molecular Genetics No specific changes.

Prognosis Benign lesion, with tendency to spontaneous regression.

Differential Diagnosis *(1) Papillary intralymphatic angioendothelioma:* it lacks the typical biphasic pattern and is poorly circumscribed. *(2) Retiform hemangioendothelioma:* it lacks the typical biphasic appearance and is larger and poorly circumscribed as compared to hobnail hemangioma. *(3) Angiosarcoma:* lacks the biphasic pattern and shows marked nuclear atypia of endothelial cells. *(4) Postradiation atypical vascular lesions:* The clinical history of exposure to radiation is essential for its diagnosis. *(5) Acquired progressive lymphangioma:* hobnail endothelium is absent, as well as hemosiderin granules and extravasated erythrocytes. *(6) Kaposi sarcoma:* it lacks the biphasic pattern, hobnail endothelium, and intravascular papillae.

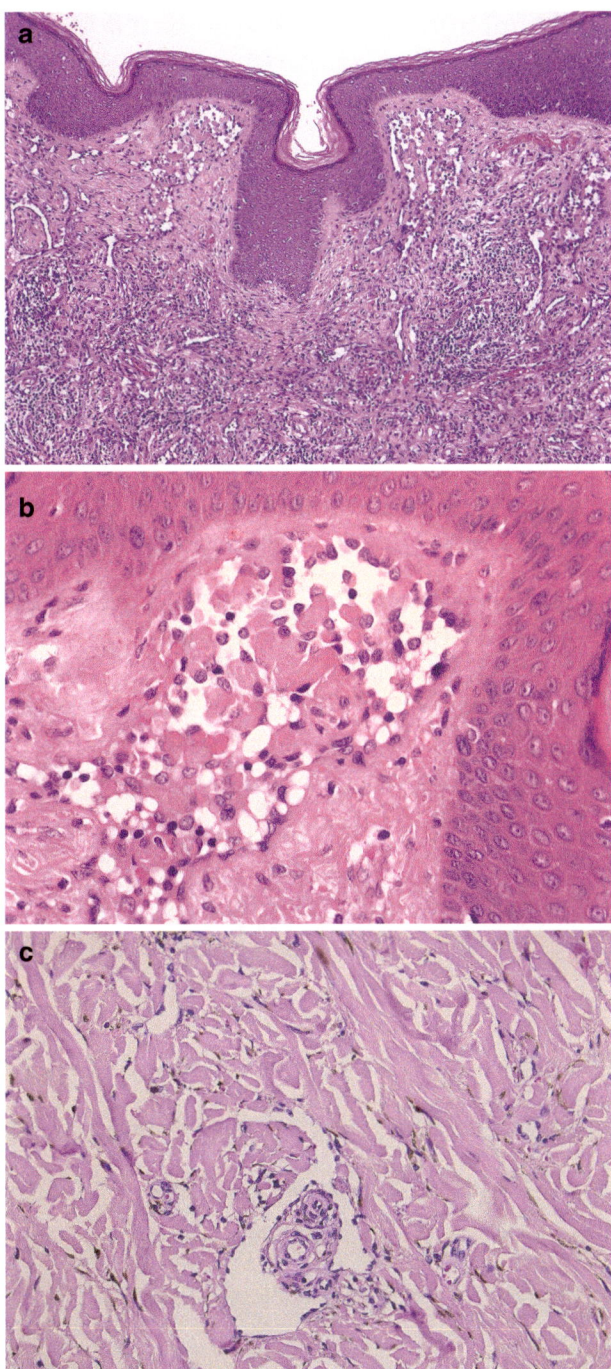

Fig. 2.34 Hobnail hemangioma from the back of a 23-year-old female at low- (**a**) and high-power fields (**b**) (HE-stained section) and deep part (**c**). Note the hobnail aspect of the superficial vessels, and the more dissecting pattern of the deeper ones

Papillary Intralymphatic Angioendothelioma (PILA) (Dabska Tumor) (Fig. 2.35)

Definition PILA is considered a rare, locally aggressive, rarely metastasizing vascular lesion, characterized by lymphatic or vascular-like channels and papillary endothelial proliferation.

Age at Presentation Infants and children > adults (40%).

Gender No sex predilection.

Localization Superficial soft tissues. No site preferred. Rare cases in deep soft tissues, bones, and spleen.

Histology Ill-defined, cavernous vascular spaces are seen, in addition to more slit-like spaces with intraluminal papillary tufts with a hobnail endothelium (Fig. 2.36a, b).

Immunohistochemistry CD31, ERG, and D2-40 are expressed, consistent with a lymphatic phenotype. CD34 may be focally expressed.

Molecular Genetics No specific change.

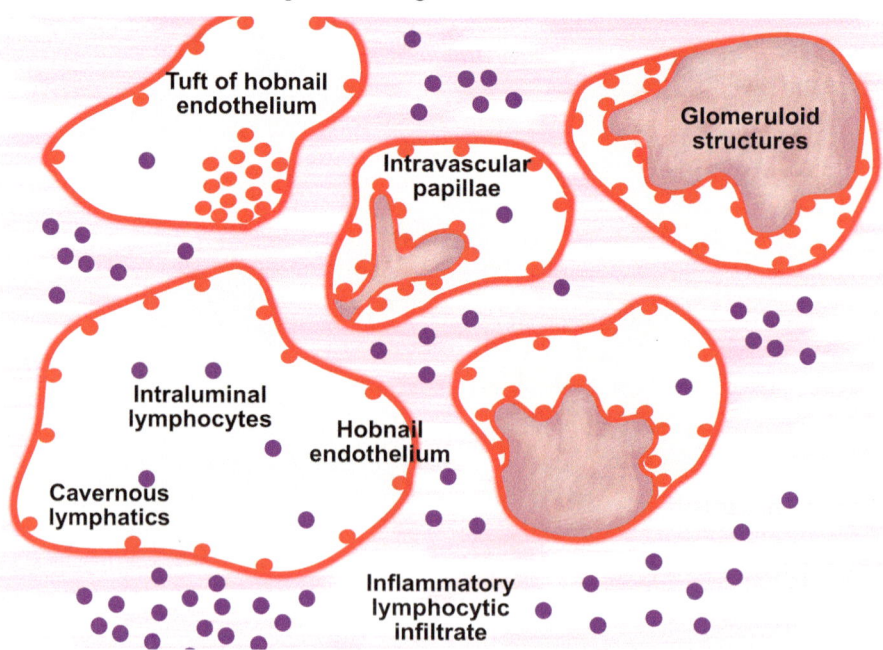

Fig. 2.35 Schematic representation of papillary intralymphatic angioendothelioma (PILA) (Dabska tumor)

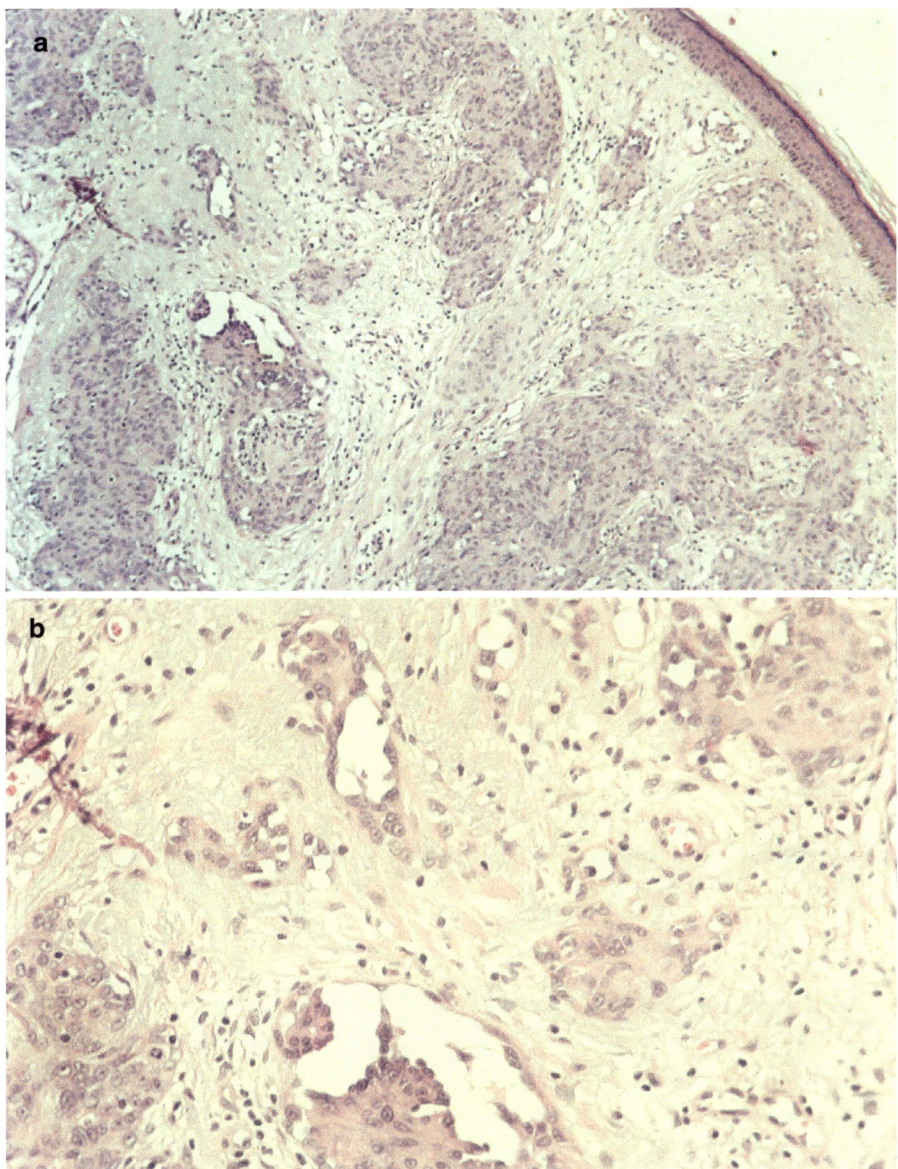

Fig. 2.36 Papillary intralymphatic angioendothelioma (PILA) (Dabska tumor) from the nose of an 81-year-old male at low- (a) and high-power fields (b) (HE-stained section), showing the prominent intravascular tufts

Prognosis There is disagreement on its biological potential. Wide excision should be curative, but close follow-up is recommended, due to lymph node metastasis reported in a minority of cases.

Acquired Elastotic Hemangioma (Fig. 2.37)

Definition Cutaneous vascular lesion, typically occurring on the forearm of elderly women, arising in the setting of sun-damaged skin.

Age at Presentation Adults >50, elderly patients.

Gender Women > men.

Localization Forearm (dorsal side) > other areas of sun-exposed skin.

Clinical Course Asymptomatic erythematous plaque, with irregular borders, mainly localized in the forearm.

Histology Band-like proliferation of dilated vessels located in the reticular dermis, associated with solar elastosis. The endothelial cells have a hobnail aspect and are not atypical. The vascular proliferation is separated by the overlying epidermis, by a grenz zone (Fig. 2.38a, b).

Immunohistochemistry A prominent rimming of alpha-SMA positive cells is always present (Fig. 2.38c, d).

Molecular Genetics No associated change.

Prognosis Excision is curative.

Differential Diagnosis The clinical diagnosis is often suggestive of basal cell carcinoma. Histology is diagnostic.

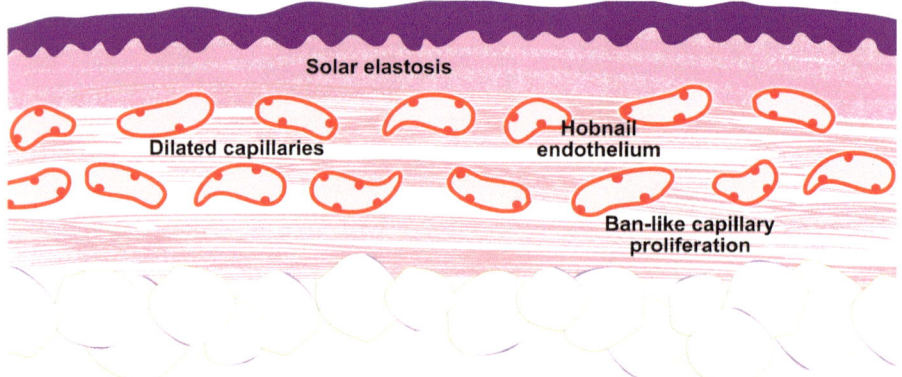

Fig. 2.37 Schematic representation of acquired elastotic hemangioma

Fig. 2.38 Acquired elastotic hemangioma from a pink plaque on the forearm of a 77-year-old female at low- (**a**) and high-power fields (**b**) (HE-stained section); immunohistochemistry for SMA (**c**) and CD31 (**d**). The band-like appearance is clear

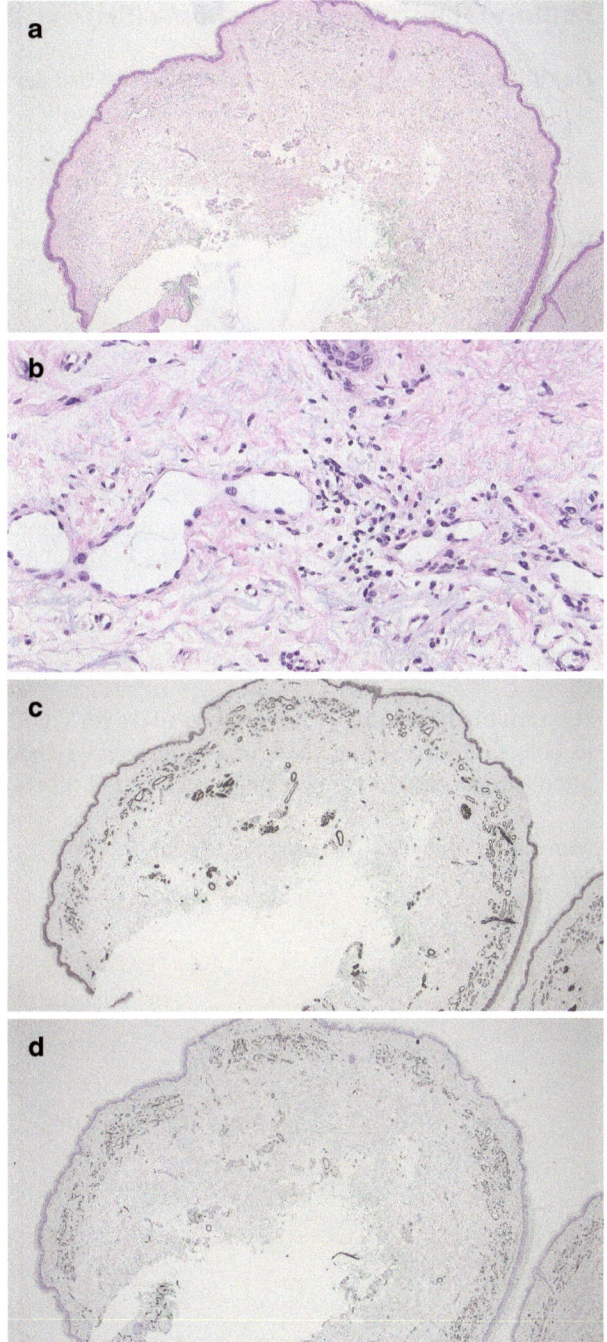

Retiform Hemangioendothelioma (RH) (Fig. 2.39)

Definition RH is a rare intermediate-grade vascular lesion mainly involving the skin and subcutaneous tissue of the distal extremities.

Age at Presentation Young adults > children > infants.

Gender No sex predilection.

Localization Extremities.

Clinical Course RH often presents with an asymptomatic slow-growing solitary nodule or plaque. Multiple lesions are rare.

Histology The whole dermis is infiltrated by branching compressed vascular structures, lined by prominent hobnail endothelial cells, with hyperchromatic but not atypical nuclei, protruding into the lumen ("tombstone"). The pattern mimics the rete testis. Small papillae may be present inside the lumen of branching vessels. Sheets or cords of spindle endothelial cells are focally found. Mitoses are rare. A dense lymphocytic infiltrate, outside and inside the vessels, is often present. Hemosiderin granules are frequent in the perivascular sclerotic dermis (Fig. 2.40a, b).

Immunohistochemistry Immunoreactivity for CD31, ERG, and CD34 is diffuse in both the hobnail endothelium and in spindle endothelial cells. Alpha-SMA is often lacking around the branching vessels. D2-40 immunostaining can be seen.

Molecular Genetics No diagnostic change.

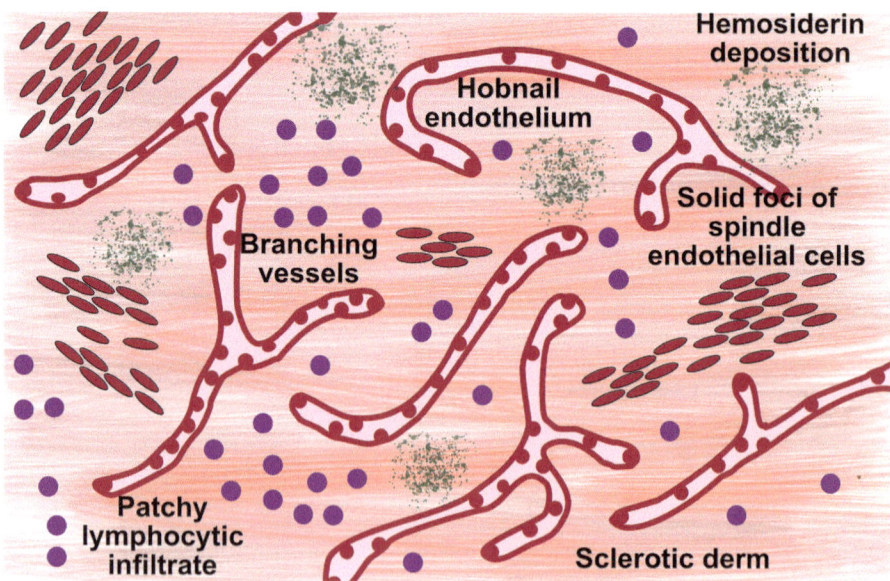

Fig. 2.39 Schematic representation of retiform hemangioendothelioma

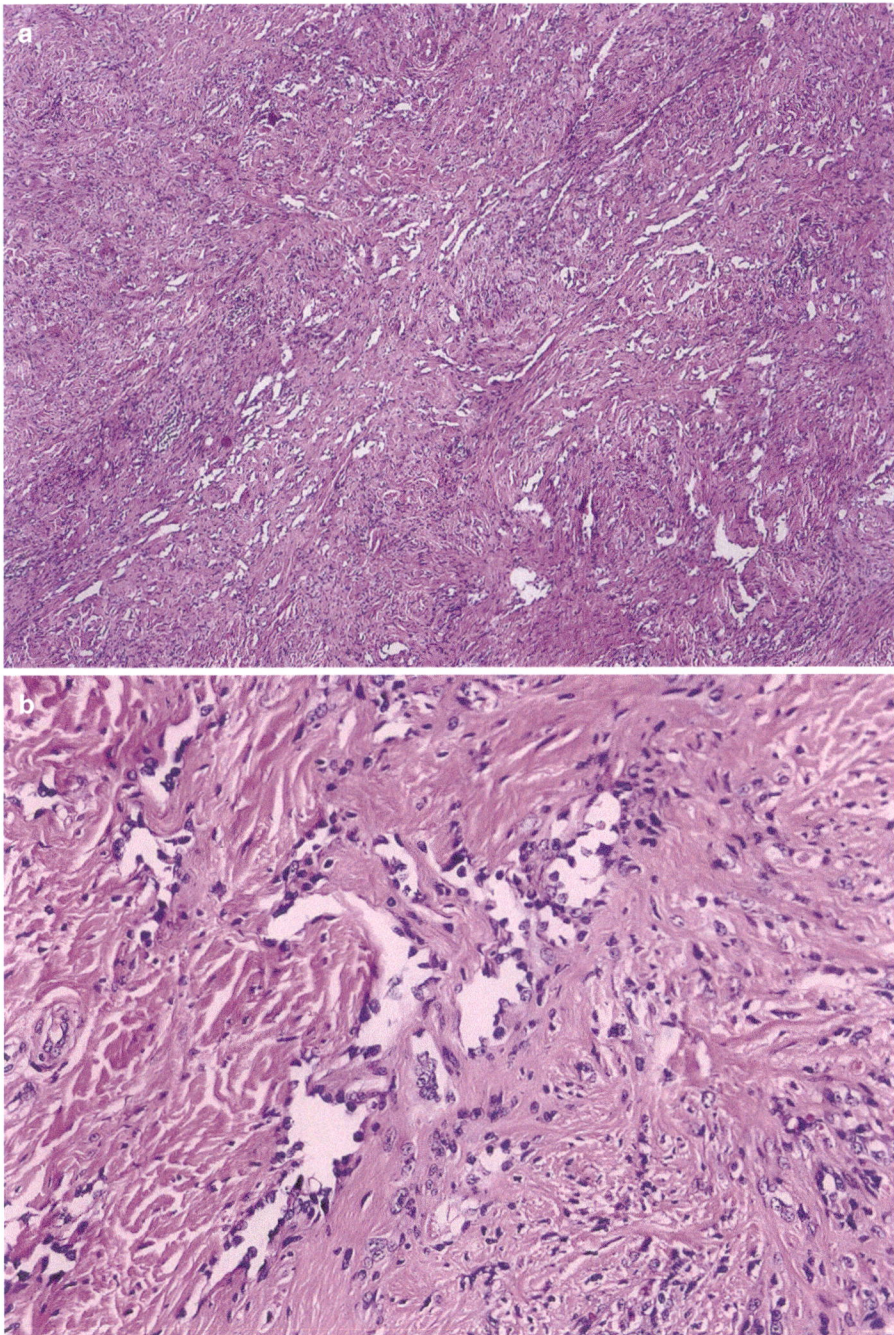

Fig. 2.40 Retiform hemangioendothelioma from the subcutis dorsum of the foot in a 31-year-old female at low- (**a**) and high-power fields (**b**) (HE-stained section). Note the retiform architecture and the hobnail apperance of the endothelium

Prognosis RH is characterized by frequent local recurrences but a very low metastatic rate. In very rare cases, RH may show an aggressive clinical course.

Differential Diagnosis *(1)* *PILA:* the presence of dilated lymphangioma-like vessels associated with abundant intraluminal papillae favors the diagnosis of PILA. *(2)* *Angiosarcoma:* endothelial multilayering and marked nuclear atypia, associated with mitoses, are in favor of the diagnosis of angiosarcoma. The location in the extremities and the young age are very unusual for angiosarcoma. *(3)* *Hobnail hemangioma:* a small, superficial, symmetric lesion with pushing margins and the restriction of hobnail endothelium to the superficial vessels favor the diagnosis of hobnail hemangioma. In RH, the hobnail feature is diffuse to the whole lesion.

Composite Hemangioendothelioma (CH)

Definition Extremely rare mixed vascular tumor of intermediate malignancy, characterized by a high recurrence rate, a rare metastatic potential, and by the possible progression to angiosarcoma following multiple recurrences.

Age at Presentation Early adulthood > children > congenital.

Gender No gender predilection.

Localization Distal extremities > oral cavity.

Clinical Course May arise as an isolated lesion or in the setting of lymphedema or Maffucci syndrome. The lesions are cutaneous or subcutaneous. Less frequently, CH may arise in the oral mucosa.

Macroscopy A cutaneous or subcutaneous nodule with infiltrative margins.

Histology The histological picture is characterized by the presence of two or more vascular tumors within the same lesion, including the association of retiform hemangioendothelioma, epithelioid and spindle cell hemangioma, or even angiosarcoma.

Immunohistochemistry Expression of CD31 and ERG. In very rare cases, nests of epithelioid cells with expression of neuro-endocrine have been reported.

Molecular Genetics No specific changes.

Prognosis The clinical behavior varies from one case to another case, ranging from a benign lesion without recurrence after surgery to tumors with high recurrence rate and metastatic potential.

Differential Diagnosis The combination of multiple (at least two) tumor patterns allows the distinction of CH from RH, epithelioid hemangioendothelioma, and low-grade angiosarcoma.

Post-irradiation Atypical Vascular Lesions (AVL) (Fig. 2.41)

Definition Skin-related vasoformative lesion arising after radiation therapy for diverse indications. Typically occurring in the irradiated skin of female patients after breast-conserving surgery or mastectomy. AVL presents a relatively short interval time between radiation and its clinical presentation (median latency 3–8 years).

Age at Presentation Any age. All changes or lesions occurring after 3 years from radiotherapy in irradiated skin should pose suspicion and be further investigated. However, female patients in their late fifties and with history of breast carcinoma are most frequently encountered.

Gender Mostly female patients, depending on the clinical setting.

Localization Skin of the irradiated field such as breast, axilla, or chest wall. However, cases in the scalp or in the larynx after irradiation for squamous cell

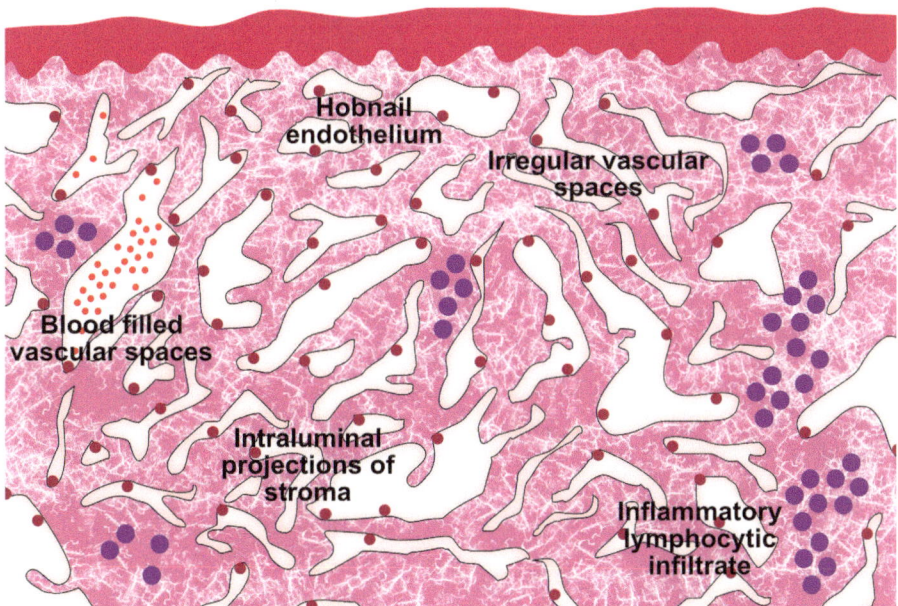

Fig. 2.41 Schematic representation of post-irradiation atypical vascular lesions (AVL)

carcinoma or hypothalamic pilocytic astrocytoma, respectively, have been documented as well.

Clinical Course Indolent clinical course. Characterized by slowly growing solitary or multiple lesions, small in size (generally not >5 mm in diameter) and with sharp margins.

Macroscopy Circumscribed reddish-brown or purple-blue papules. Less frequently AVL presents as a plaque, nodule, or vesicle. Lesions of 20 mm or larger are infrequent.

Histology At low-power magnification, the lesion is relatively well circumscribed, symmetrical, located in the superficial-mid dermis, and often wedge shaped. Extension to the deep dermis is uncommon. At higher magnification, a proliferation of delicate vascular spaces with a tiny wall and irregular to angulated shape is observed. Sometimes focal anastomoses can be present as well. The lining endothelium shows a very bland cytology and lacks a multilayering or architectural complexity. Hobnailing with hyperchromatic not atypical nuclei can be observed (Fig. 2.42). AVL is consistently mitotically inactive. Tiny intraluminal projections of stroma lined by endothelium are frequently observed in the lumen of ectatic vessels. Blood-filled vascular spaces are less frequently observed; red blood

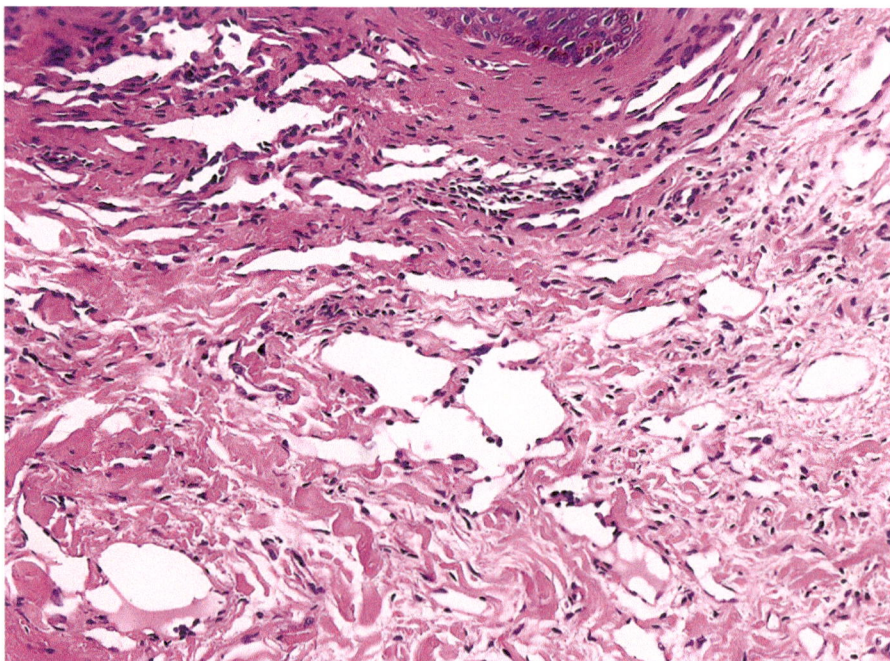

Fig. 2.42 Post-irradiation AVL, occurring in a female of 64 years old, who was treated by radio-therapy for a breast carcinoma 4 years ago (HE-stained section). Note the superficial dilated vascular spaces with the hobnail endothelium

cells extravasation is absent. AVL is frequently associated with a sparse to moderate chronic inflammatory infiltrate. Occasionally some lesions may appear focally less circumscribed with more inter-anastomosing and pseudo-infiltrative growth pattern with dermal dissection, mimicking angiosarcoma.

Variants Two variants are recognized depending on the immunohistochemical expression of podoplanin (D2-40): lymphatic and vascular. The clinical relevance of this distinction is debated.

Immunohistochemistry CD31 and ERG are expressed. Podoplanin is usually positive in the lymphatic variant, which on occasion may show focal expression of CD34. Pericytic markers show a complete circular layer in the vascular variant, while in the lymphatic variant it is incomplete.

Molecular Genetics No specific molecular hallmarks.

Prognosis AVL is a benign lesion for which, if clinically feasible, surgical resection with free margins is curative. In 15–30% of the cases, recurrence has been reported either as a consequence of incomplete resection or as a new lesion arising within the same radiation field. Cases of malignant progression and coexistence with post-irradiation sarcoma have rarely been reported. Therefore, appropriate sampling while grossing and regular clinical follow-up are important in the management of AVL.

Differential Diagnosis The main differential diagnosis is with *post-irradiation angiosarcoma*. Architectural features that favor angiosarcoma include lack of circumscription, prominent inter-anastomosing vessels, marked dermal collagen dissection, presence of infiltration in the subcutaneous tissue, marked multilayering of endothelial cells, and inflammation. The presence of nuclear atypia with hobnailing, prominent nucleoli, and mitotic activity represent the cytological features favoring the diagnosis of angiosarcoma (Fig. 2.43a). However, angiosarcomas can show very subtle histological changes especially at the periphery, rendering the differential diagnosis with AVL extremely challenging, especially in case of tiny diagnostic biopsies. In this regard, the knowledge that over 90% of post-irradiation angiosarcomas harbor amplification of the *C-MYC* gene and show protein expression at nuclear level can represent a useful diagnostic aid to solve the differential diagnosis (Fig. 2.43c). Indeed, AVL lacks *C-MYC* amplification and only occasionally shows weak nuclear C-MYC staining by immunohistochemistry. Sometimes sporadic C-MYC expression can be observed also in benign vessels present in irradiated skin biopsies. Therefore, in situ hybridization techniques should be used as reflex test to check the *C-MYC* gene status in difficult cases.

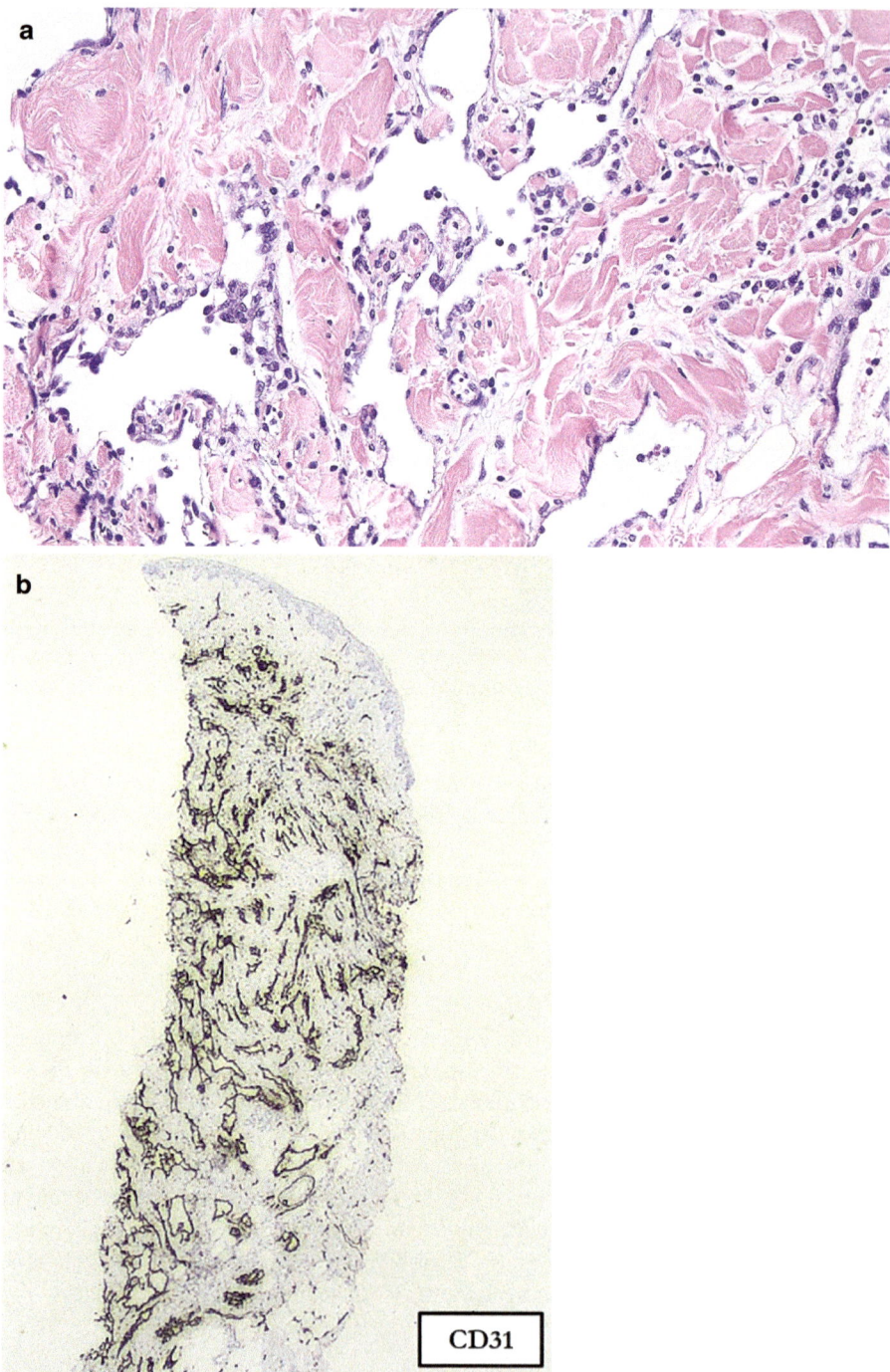

Fig. 2.43 Post-irradiation angiosarcoma in a 67-years–old female, treated 9 years ago by radiotherapy for a breast carcinoma. Note the dissecting pattern and the piling up of atypical endothelial cells (a) (HE-stained section) immunochemisrty for CD31 (b) and C-MYC (c), showing the prominent nuclear C-MYC staining

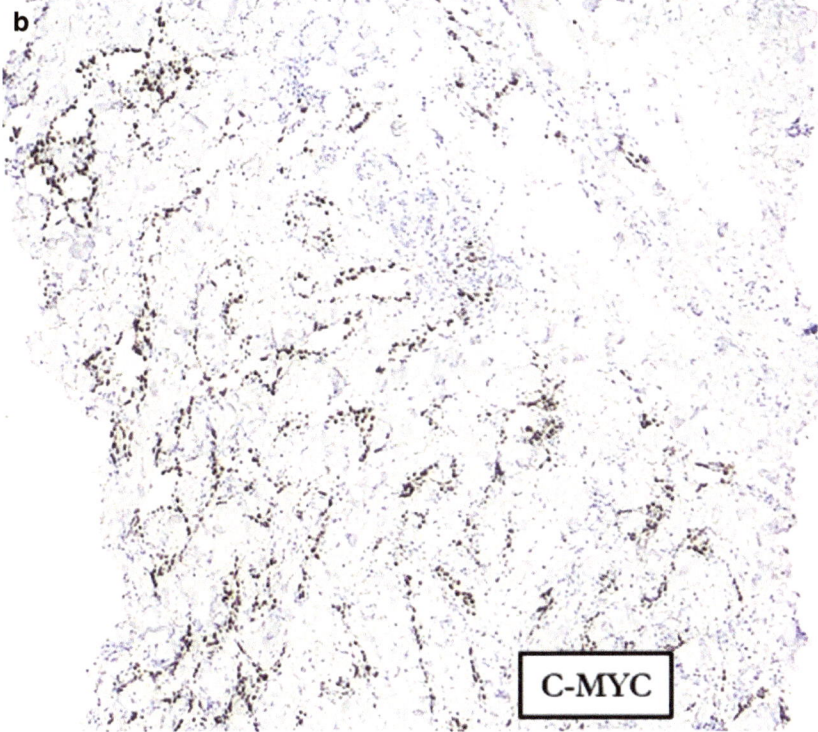

Fig. 2.43 (continued)

Vascular Tumors with Spindle Cell Phenotype

Spindle Cell Hemangioma (SCH) (Fig. 2.44)

Definition Previously considered a low-grade sarcoma, also misinterpreted as hemangioendothelioma, it is a benign vascular lesion characterized by a spindle cell proliferation and cavernous blood vessels.

Age at Presentation Young adults more affected. Wide age range.

Gender No sex predilection.

Localization Subcutis of distal extremities > chest wall > head and neck > oral cavity.

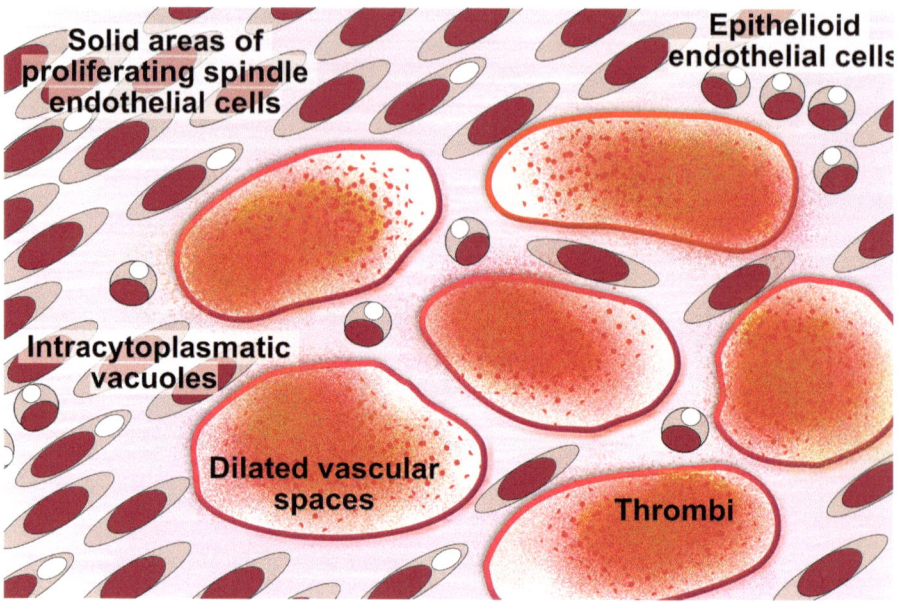

Fig. 2.44 Schematic representation of spindle cell hemangioma (SCH)

Clinical Course SCH may be sporadic or, less frequently, associated with enchondromas, in the setting of Maffucci syndrome, with Klippel-Trénaunay syndrome, congenital lymphedema, or early onset varicosites. Multiple lesions are present in half of the patients.

Macroscopy Swelling of the affected area or bluish nodules are the presenting symptoms.

Histology Well-circumscribed multiple nodular lesions, localized in the deep dermis or in the subcutaneous tissue. Nodules are composed of dilated vascular spaces, with thrombi, surrounded by solid areas of proliferating spindle to epithelioid endothelial cells with intracytoplasmic vacuoles (Fig. 2.45a–c). Intravascular growth can be seen.

Immunohistochemistry Endothelial cells show reactivity for CD31, ERG, and CD34. The more solid vacuolated cells are often alpha-SMA positive.

Molecular Genetics In about 70% of cases, *IDH1* or *IDH2* mutations are present.

Prognosis Conservative surgical excision is the preferred treatment. In +/− 60% of cases, lesions 'recur' due to intravascular multifocal growth.

Fig. 2.45 Spindle cell hemangioma (SCH) from a 35-year-old male with Maffucci syndrome at low- (**a**) and high-power fields (**b**) and with vacuoles (**c**) (HE-stained section). Note the combination of dilated vessels with spindle cells that can show vacuolisation

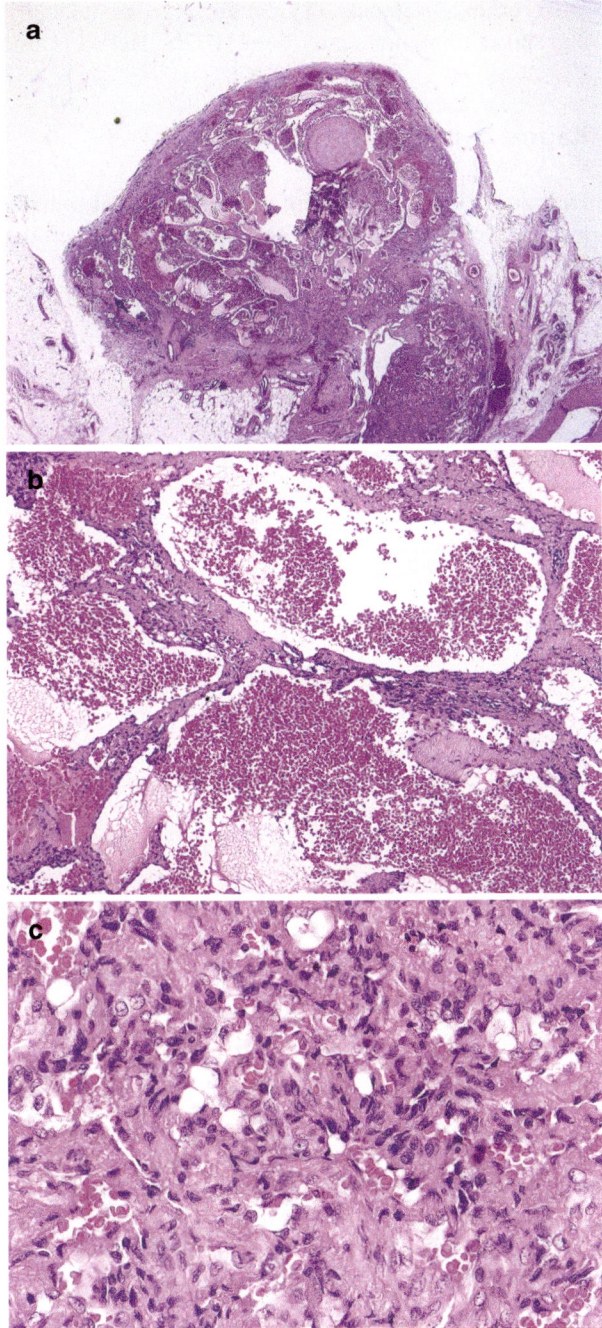

Differential Diagnosis (1) *Kaposi sarcoma*: it lacks the cavernous vascular spaces and shows immunoreactivity for HHV8. HHV8 is always negative in SCH.

Kaposi Sarcoma (KS) (Fig. 2.46)

Definition Lesion of intermediate biological potential, representing a multifocal human herpesvirus 8 (HHV8)-induced vascular proliferation.

Age at Presentation Adults, except the aggressive subtype of the African-endemic KS that presents in children.

Gender Males predominate (15/1) in classical KS and in African-endemic KS.

Localization Cutaneous lesions are mainly localized in distal extremities, mainly feet. Extracutaneous localizations include lymph nodes, the gastrointestinal tract, and the lungs.

Clinical Course In all the clinical variants, KS is characterized by three clinical-pathological stages: *(1) the patch stage,* characterized by bluish macules;

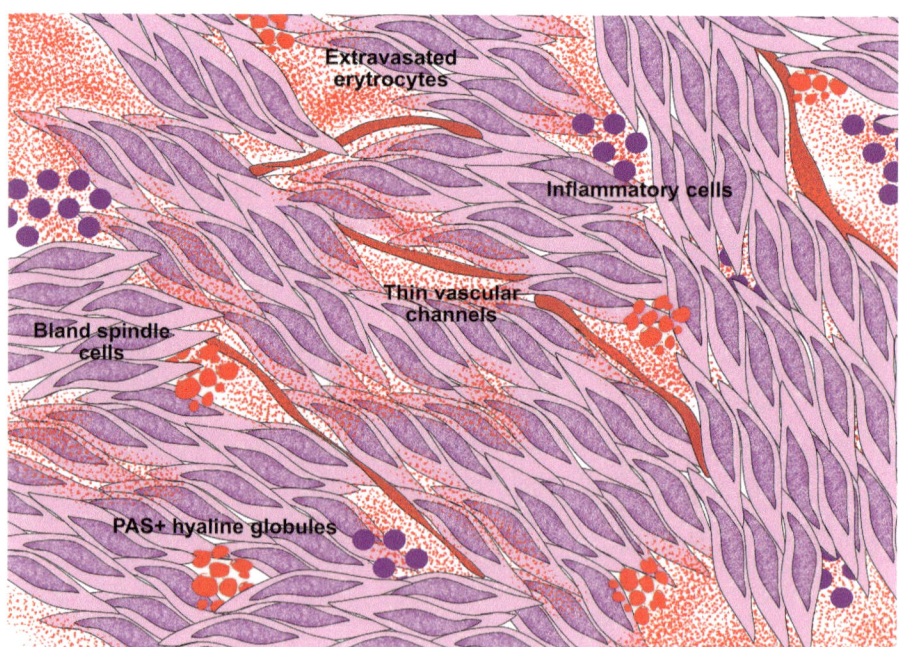

Fig. 2.46 Schematic representation of Kaposi sarcoma (KS)

(2) the plaque stage, in which macules become elevated and progress to plaques; and *(3) the nodular stage,* in which lesions become nodular.

Histology Irregular thin vascular channels, associated with a proliferation of bland spindle cells containing intracellular PAS+ hyaline globules, characterize all subtypes of KS. In the *patch stage* (Fig. 2.47), the vascular component is dominant. Thin vascular channels, sometimes lymphangioma-like, dissect the collagen fibers of the superficial and reticular dermis. Adnexal structures may be completely encircled by the thin-walled vessels and isolated from the surrounding dermis, giving rise to the "promontory sign." In between the vessels, some bland spindle cells admixed with some inflammatory cells may be seen. In *the plaque stage* (Fig. 2.48a, b), the whole reticular dermis is infiltrated by the thin vessels and by the spindle cells, which may extend into the subcutaneous fat. In this stage, spindle cells represent the dominating component of KS. Lymphocytes, plasma cells, extravasated red blood cells, hemosiderin granules, and hyaline globules complete the histological picture. *Nodular KS* (Fig. 2.49a, b) is characterized by a marked predominance of spindle cells, arranged in fascicles, with intermingled thin slit-like vascular spaces containing extravasated erythrocytes . Mitoses and hyaline globules (Fig. 2.49c) are frequent. *Lymph node involvement from KS* starts with few irregular vessels extending from the subcapsular sinus along the cortical and medullary sinuses, ending with the complete invasion of the lymph node.

Variants Four main clinical variants of KS are recognized: *(1) Classical KS:* it affects elderly subjects from the East Europe or Mediterranean area, including the island of Sardinia. Lesions are preferentially localized in feet. Mucosal or visceral involvement is seen in a minority of patients. *(2) African endemic KS:* it may present in three clinical subtypes: (a) an aggressive and often fatal form, presenting in children with systemic lymphadenopathy; (b) an aggressive cutaneous variant, often associated with bone involvement; (c) a cutaneous indolent form, resembling classical KS. *(3) Iatrogenic KS:* it occurs as a consequence of the use of immunosuppressive drugs in patients who underwent transplantation. The clinical course ranges from a disseminated aggressive disease to an indolent skin lesion that may regress, halting the use of immunosuppressive drugs. *(4) AIDS-related KS:* it is a typical form affecting homosexual men with AIDS. The clinical course ranges from an indolent disease to a very aggressive form, characterized by cutaneous and visceral involvement.

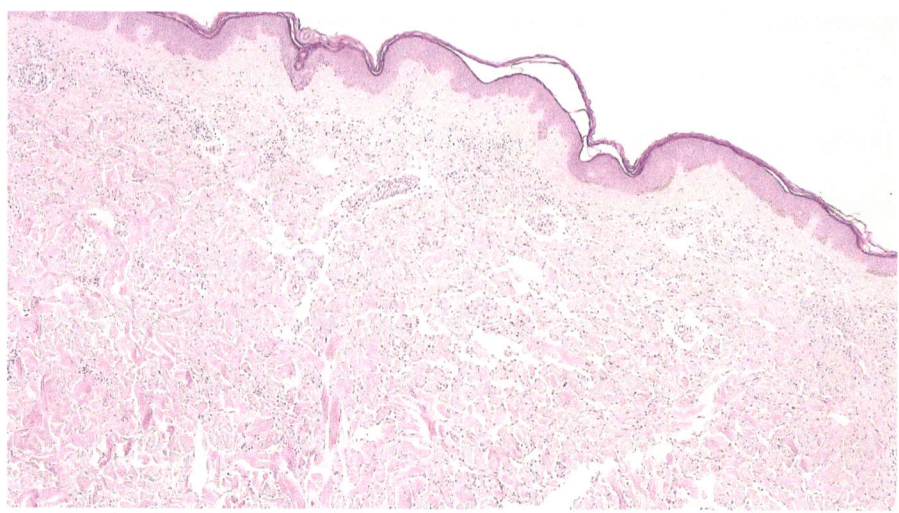

Fig. 2.47 Patch stage of Kaposi sarcoma from the pink lesions in the groin of a 42-year HIV+ male. Dilated vessels predominate

Immunohistochemistry Spindle and endothelial cells are immunoreactive to CD34 (Fig. 2.50a), CD31, ERG, D2-40 (Fig. 2.50b), and nuclear granular HHV8 (Fig. 2.50c, d). The latter may be very weak in the patch stage.

Molecular Genetics No diagnostic utility.

Prognosis It depends on the patient's immunocompetence.

Differential Diagnosis (1) *Dermatitis:* the patch stage of KS may show so subtle changes that may mimic a simple inflammatory pattern. (2) *Hobnail hemangioma*: the finding of a spindle cell component and of abundant plasma cells favors KS. (3) *Angiosarcoma*: the absence of marked atypia and endothelial multilayering favors the diagnosis of KS. HHV8 is nearly always negative in angiosarcoma.

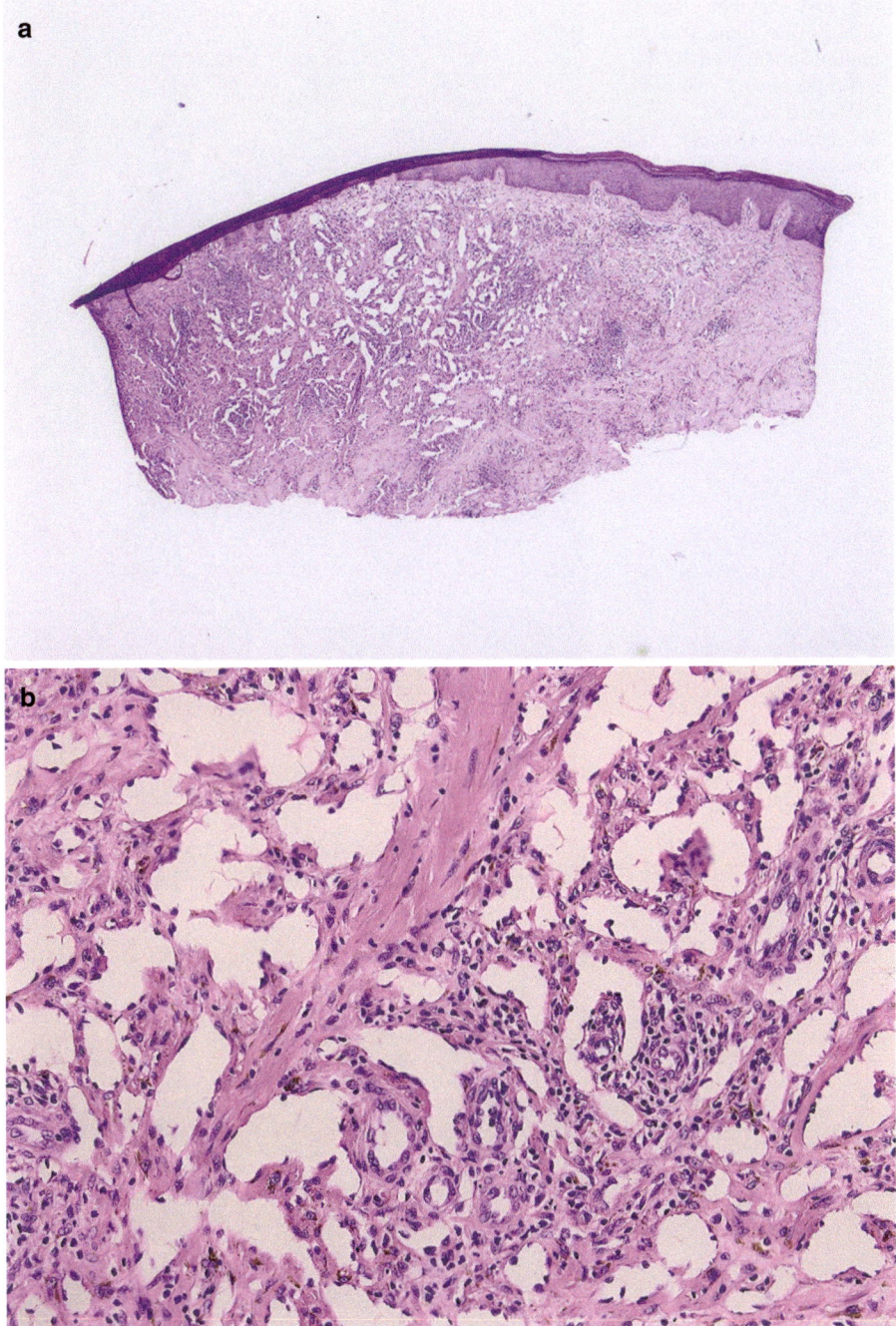

Fig. 2.48 Plaque stage of Kaposi sarcoma from a 74-year-old, HIV−, Turkish male presenting as slowly growing pink plaques on lower legs since 10 years at low- (**a**) and high-power fields with promontory signs (**b**) (HE-stained section)

Fig. 2.49 Nodular stage of Kaposi sarcoma from multiple nodules on the lower leg of a 67-year-old HIV− male at low- (**a**), medium- (**b**), and high-power fields (**c**) and with globules (HE-stained section)

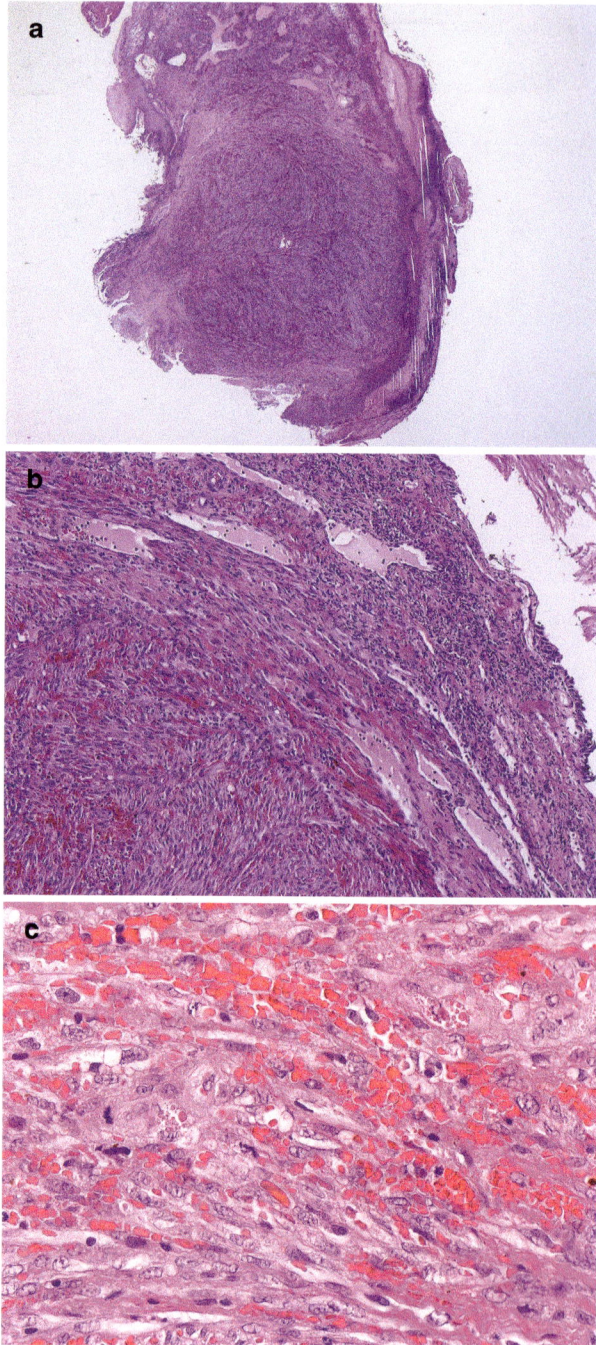

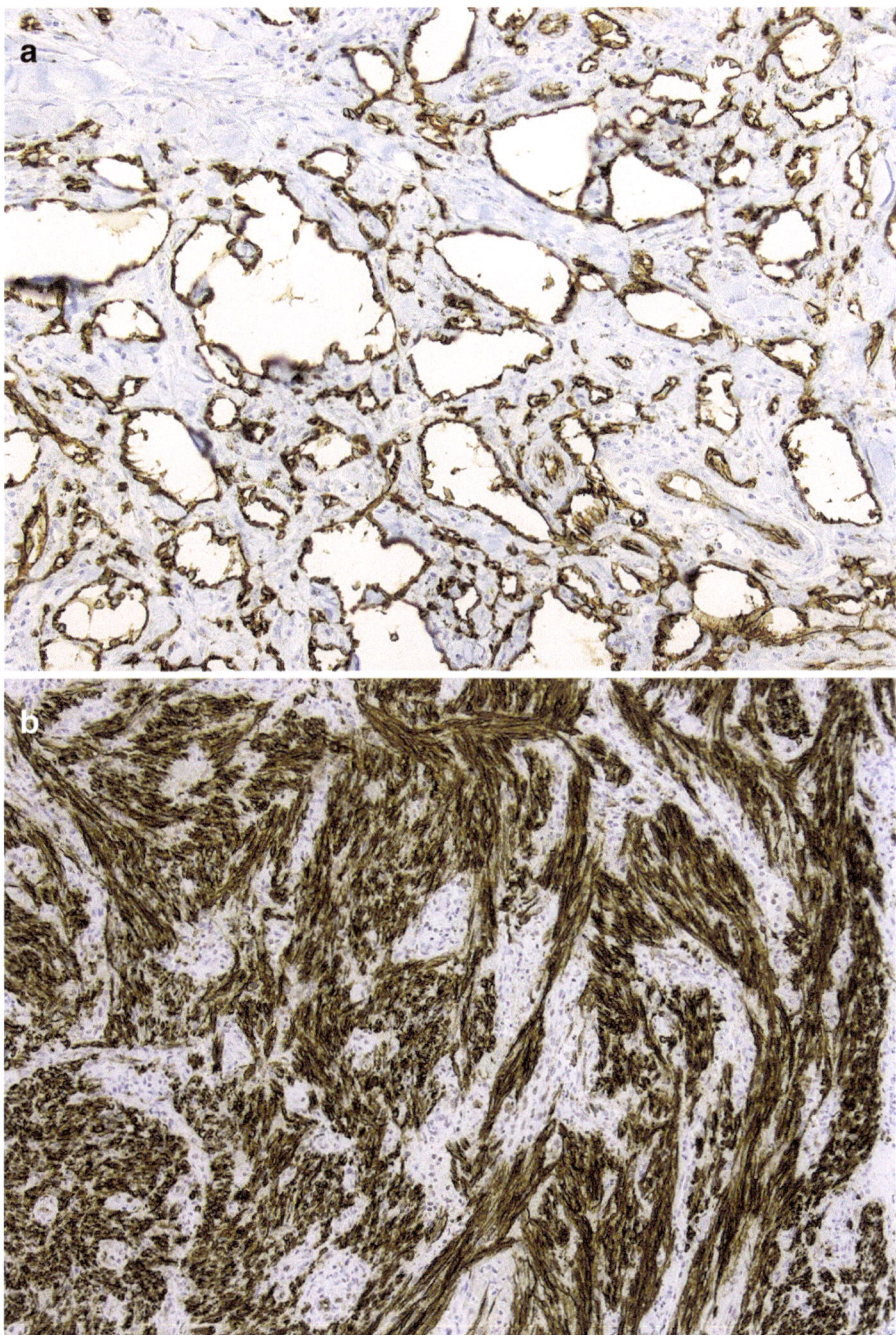

Fig. 2.50 Immunohistochemistry for CD34 in the plaque stage of Kaposi sarcoma (**a**) (see also Fig. 2.48); immunohistochemistry for D2-40 of nodular stage of Kaposi sarcoma (**b**) (see also Fig. 2.49); immunohistochemistry for HHV8 in patch stage (**c**) (see also Fig. 2.47) and nodular stage (**d**) (see also Fig. 2.49) of Kaposi sarcoma

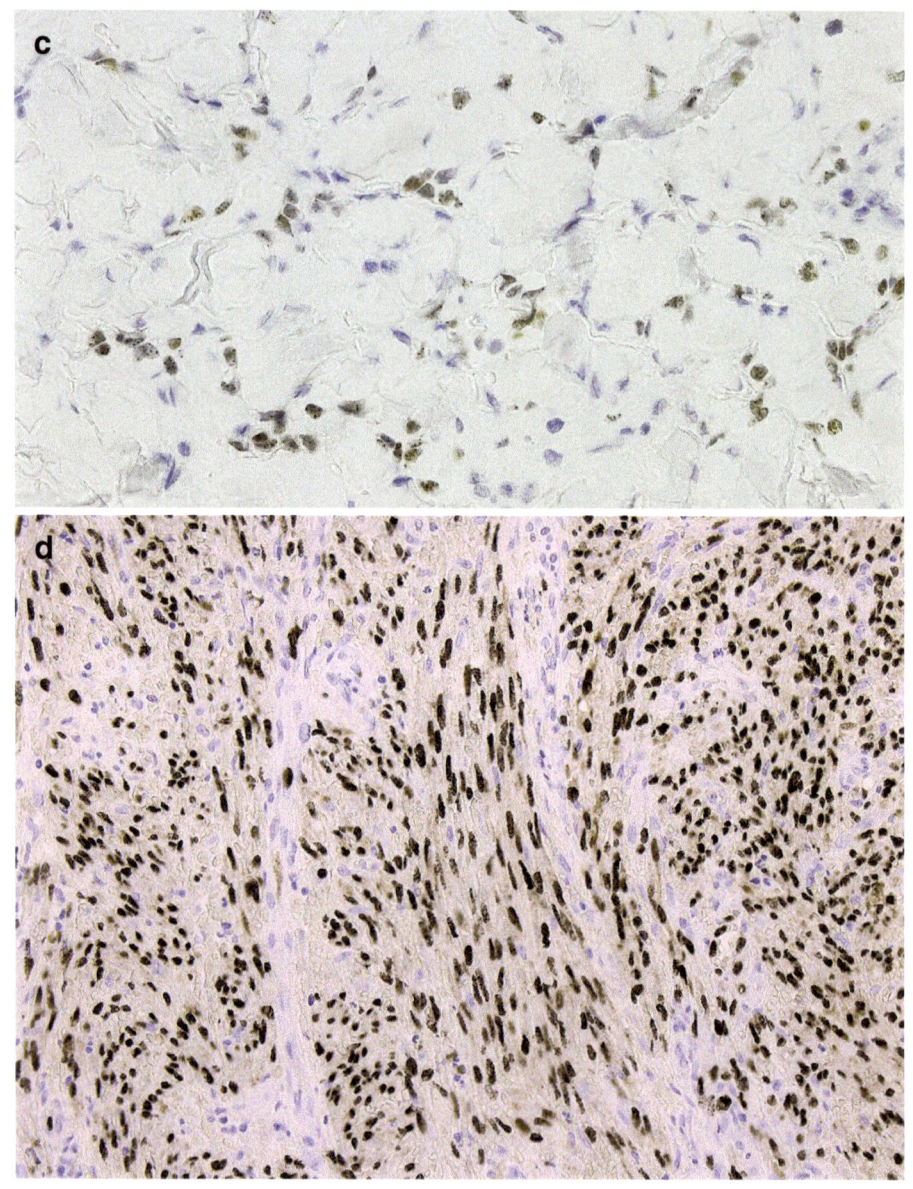

Fig. 2.50 (continued)

Kaposiform Hemangioendothelioma (Fig. 2.51)

Definition A rare vascular tumor, mainly in children, characterized by dense lobules of capillaries and spindled cells, associated with dilated lymphatic vessels.

Age at Presentation Infancy > young adults > adults (rare).

Localization Extremities > retroperitoneum > head and neck (rare). Sometimes multifocal.

Clinical Course Deep lesions of the lips present as an indurated nodule. Clinical presentation of retroperitoneal lesions depends on the site of origin: abdominal distension, gastrointestinal bleeding, obstruction, and jaundice are the most frequent symptoms. Fifty percent of patients develop Kabasach-Merritt syndrome, due to platelet trapping within proliferating vascular structures, ending with severe thrombocytopenia. Association with lymphangiomatosis is reported in one of five cases.

Macroscopy Retroperitoneal tumors appear at surgery as a highly infiltrative mass, extending into the abdominal wall and retroperitoneal and abdominal organs. Deep tumors of the limbs show a similar infiltrative tendency.

Histology Large lobules ("canon balls") of bland spindle cells with abundant cytoplasm, separated by slit-like spaces containing red blood cells. At the periphery of the lobules, dilated lymphatics and capillaries with microthrombi are often found (Fig. 2.52a, b).

Immunohistochemistry CD31 and ERG are expressed. D2-40 can be positive in the lobules. GLUT-1 is negative. Alpha-SMA is negative in the spindle cells lobules.

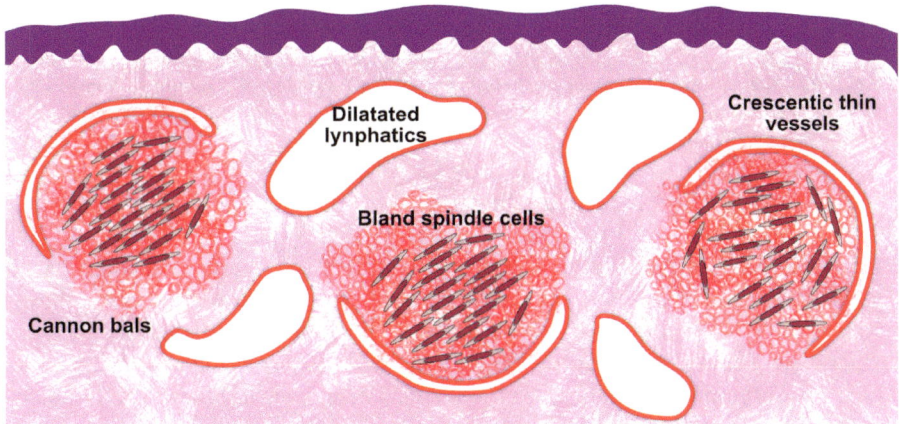

Fig. 2.51 Schematic representation of Kaposiform hemangioendothelioma

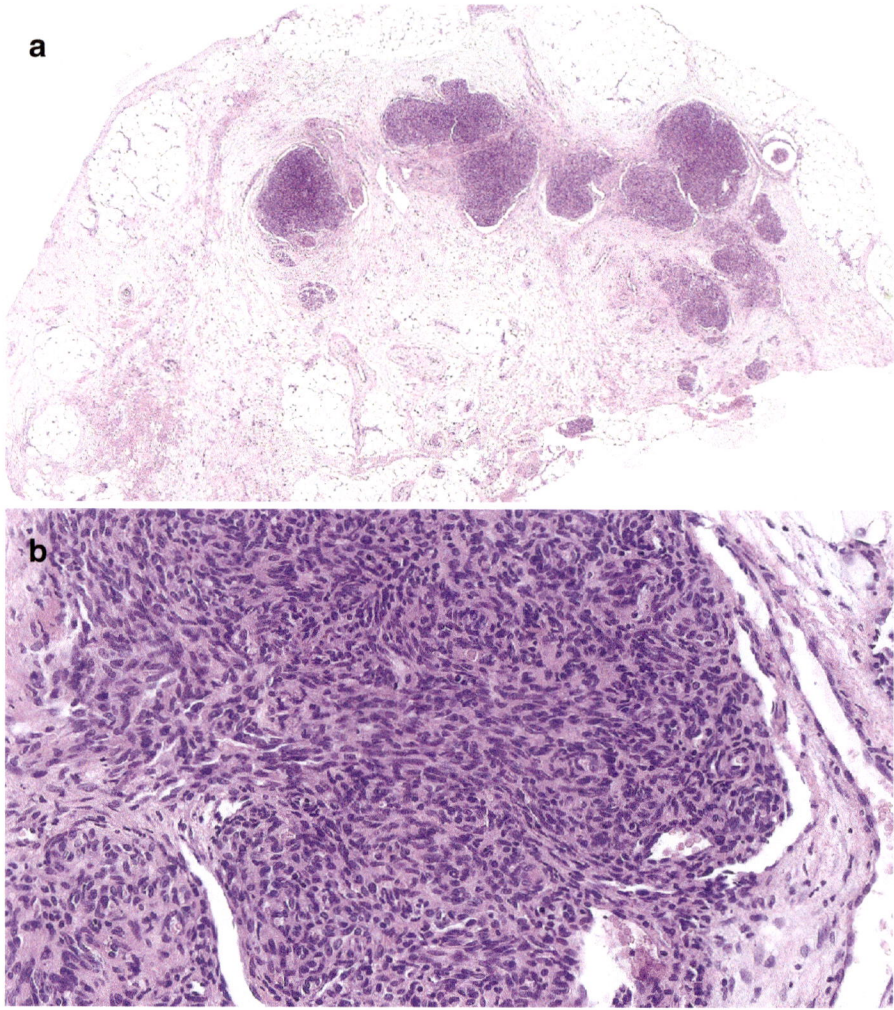

Fig. 2.52 Kaposiform hemangioendothelioma from the lower leg of a boy of 4 months old, at low- (**a**) and high-power fields (**b**) (HE-stained section). Note the 'canon-balls' of capillaries surrounded by slit-like vessels

Molecular Genetics No specific changes.

Prognosis The clinical course and the efficacy of therapy depend on the localization and the extent of thrombopenia. Retroperitoneal tumors show a considerable mortality rate. Combination chemotherapy regimens, including vincristine, show higher efficacy when compared to a surgical approach. Extension to regional lymph nodes is frequent, but "metastatic lesions" are probably rather a sign of multifocal disease.

Differential Diagnosis *(1) Kaposi sarcoma:* it is very rare in childhood. The absence of HHV8 reactivity and of a lympho-plasmocytic infiltrate favors the diagnosis of Kaposiform hemangioendothelioma.

Spindle Cell Angiosarcoma

Definition High-grade angiosarcoma characterized by a predominant or exclusive spindle cell morphology.

Age at Presentation Similar to vasoformative AS.

Gender Similar to vasoformative AS.

Localization Similar to vasoformative AS.

Clinical Course Similar to vasoformative AS.

Macroscopy Similar to vasoformative AS.

Histology Spindle cells arranged in short fascicles, with atypical hyperchromatic nuclei, intermingled with slit-like vascular channels containing erythrocytes. Blister cells, with intracytoplasmatic vacuoles may be focally detected, suggesting an endothelial origin of the undifferentiated spindle cells. At the periphery of the lesion, neoplastic vessels with markedly atypical nuclei are often found (Fig. 2.53a).

Variants A rare variant is characterized by long fascicles, with a *fibrosarcoma-like* pattern.

Immunohistochemistry Immunostaining is similar to vasoformative angiosarcoma. An antibody panel, including broad-spectrum cytokeratins, S-100 protein, CD31, and ERG should be used in the differential diagnosis with other spindle cell tumors (Fig. 2.53b, c).

Molecular Genetics Similar to vasoformative AS.

Prognosis Similar to vasoformative AS.

Differential Diagnosis (1) *Spindle cell carcinoma*; (keratin ++), (2) *spindle cell variant of atypical fibroxanthoma* (circumscribed, no vascular markers, CD10+, p53++), (3) Kaposi sarcoma (HHV8 expression).

Fig. 2.53 Spindle cell angiosarcoma from the heart in a 20-year-old male (HE-stained section) (**a**); immunohistochemistry shows positivity for CD31 (**b**) and negativity for HHV8 (**c**)

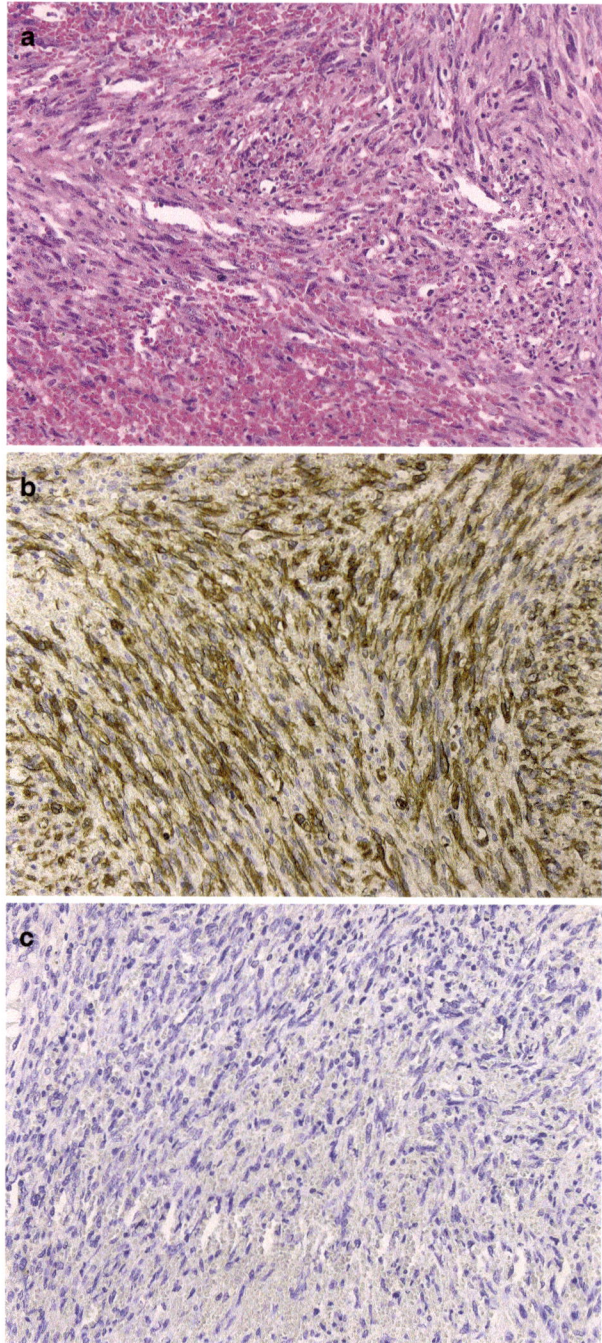

Vascular Tumors with Epithelioid Phenotype

Epithelioid Hemangioma (EH)

Definition Vasoformative vascular tumor with prominent epithelioid cells admixed with an inflammatory component, previously also labeled as angiolymphoid hyperplasia with eosinophilia.

Age at Presentation Young to middle-aged adults.

Gender No sex predilection.

Localization Head and neck (peri-auricular zone) > distal extremities > oral mucosa, penis, lymph nodes (rarely).

Clinical Course Superficial tumors present as solitary or multiple erythematous pruritic papulae or as small cutaneous nodules. Lesions arising in deep soft tissues present as nodular masses.

Histology The lesions are +/− lobular and consist of capillary-sized vessels with plump epithelioid cells with non-atypical vesicular nuclei and an intact myopericytic layer. In between, lymphoid follicles or dispersed lymphocytes and/or eosinophils can be numerous (Fig. 2.54a).

Variants A cellular variant with predilection to the bones and penis are described, with a more solid growth and nuclear pleomorphism and necrosis. They are associated with a more aggressive loco-regional growth.

Immunohistochemistry Keratin expression is usually limited but strong and diffuse expression of endothelial markers such as ERG and CD31 (Fig. 2.54b) is always present. D2-40 is negative and alpha-SMA usually decorates the perivascular cuff (Fig. 2.54c). FOSB expression is seen in about half of the classical and cellular cases.

Molecular Genetics Classical EH shows *FOS* (14q24.3) rearrangement; the cellular variant is characterized by *FOSB* (19q13.2) rearrangement.

Prognosis About a third of the lesions recur. The cellular variants may be more aggressive, but the difference between multifocal or metastatic disease is not clear.

Fig. 2.54 Epithelioid hemangioma from the toe of a 15-year-old male (HE-stained section) (**a**); immunohistochemistry shows positivity for CD31 (**b**) and for SMA (**c**)

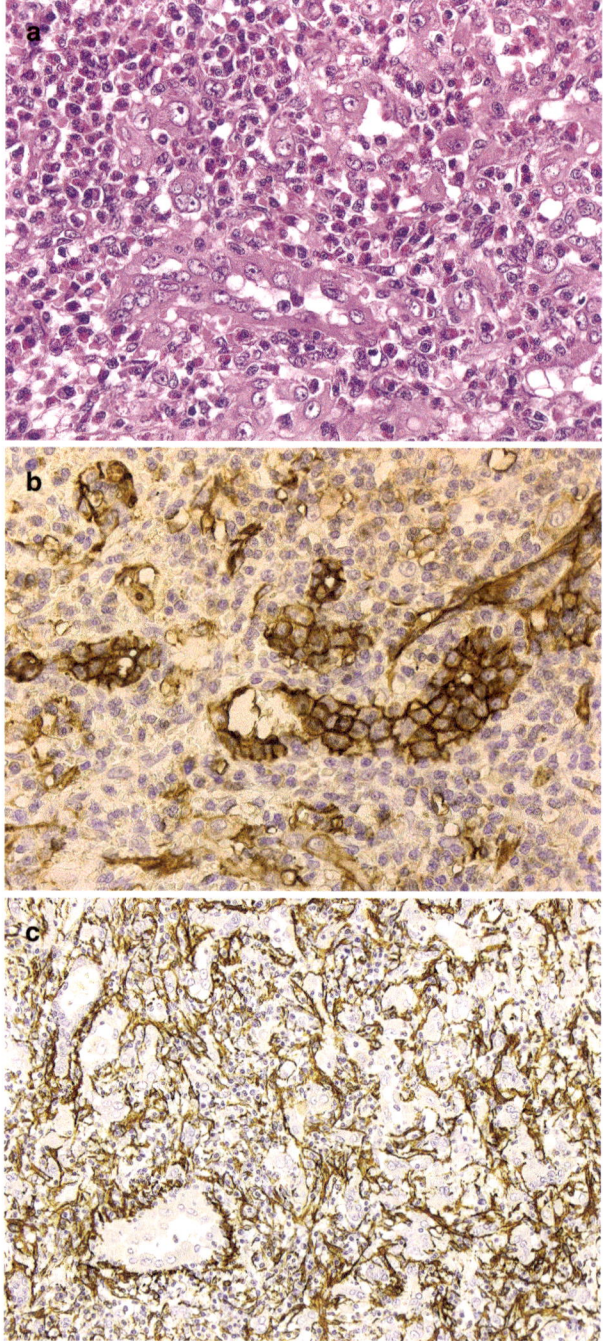

Epithelioid Angiomatous Nodule (EAN) (Fig. 2.55)

Definition Benign nodular superficial dermal vascular tumor, often exophitic, with epithelioid appearance.

Age at Presentation Young to middle-aged adults.

Gender No predilection.

Localization Distribution is wide. Cutaneous > subcutaneous > mucosal.

Clinical Course A well-circumscribed dermal nodule, <1 cm in diameter, red-blue in color. EAN has been reported even in mucosae. Cases with multiple nodules have been rarely described.

Histology Small superficial circumscribed nodule, surrounded by a hyperplastic epidermis, sometimes with a collarette. The architecture is predominantly solid and a vasoformative character may be lacking. Tumor cells are large, epithelioid, with abundant cytoplasm, frequent intracytoplasmic vacuoles, and large vesicular nuclei with prominent nucleoli. Tumor cells are arranged in solid sheets, with intermingled red blood cells. Mitotic figures can be seen, but not atypical ones (Fig. 2.56a, b).

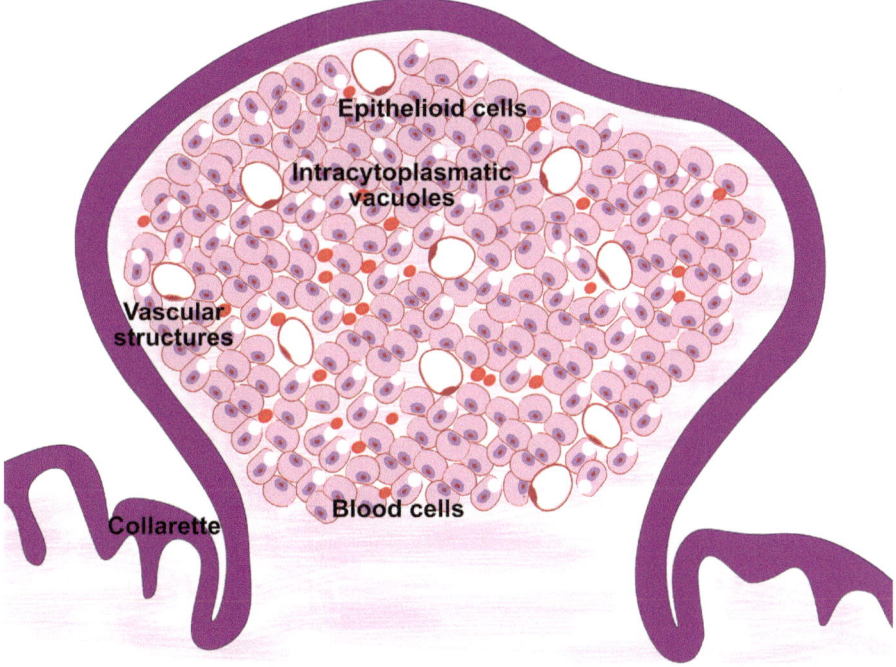

Fig. 2.55 Schematic representation of epithelioid angiomatous nodule (EAN)

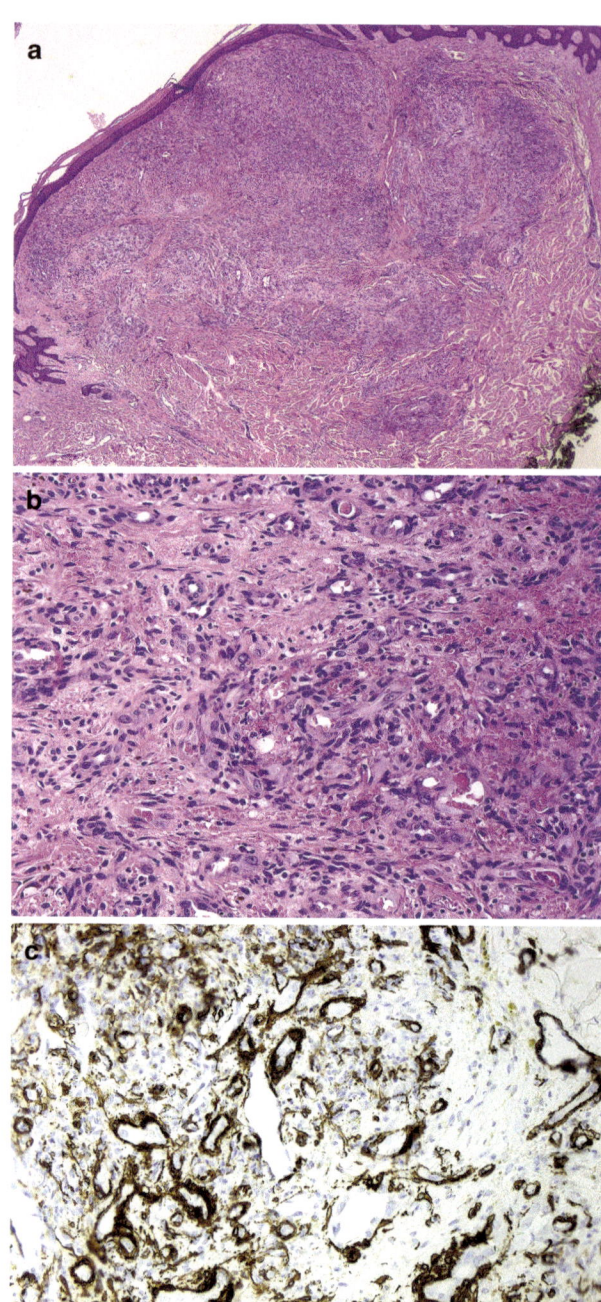

Fig. 2.56 Epithelioid angiomatous nodule (EAN) from the back of an 86-year-old male, at low- (**a**) and high-power fields (**b**) (HE-stained section); immunohistochemistry for SMA (**c**)

Immunohistochemistry Tumor cells express ERG and CD31, keratin is generally not expressed (Fig. 2.56c).

Molecular Genetics No specific changes.

Prognosis Excision is curative.

Differential Diagnosis It can show considerable overlap with *epithelioid hemangioma* and pyogenic granuloma and thus could be considered a variant of these lesions. *Epithelioid angiosarcoma:* it is characterized by a marked cytological atypia that is lacking in EAN.

Pseudomyogenic Hemangioendothelioma (PHE) (Fig. 2.57)

Definition Also known as epithelioid sarcoma-like hemangioendothelioma, PHE is an often multifocal vascular tumor of intermediate biological potential that resembles a myoid/epithelioid tumor.

Age at Presentation Young adults (< 50 years).

Gender Male predominance: M/F = 5/1.

Localization Lower extremities > arms.

Clinical Course One or multiple superficial cutaneous nodules, which tend to extend to the subcutaneous tissue, to underlying muscles (half of patients) and, occasionally, to bones.

Macroscopy Well-circumscribed nodular lesions, 1–2 cm in diameter. Variable cut surface, fibrous to fleshy.

Histology Fascicles and sheets of spindle cells with abundant eosinophilic cytoplasm, clear vesicular nuclei with prominent nucleoli. Focally, tumor cells show an abundant ground-glass cytoplasm, and a polar nucleus, with a rhabdomyoblast-like appearance. Scattered tumor cells show an epithelioid appearance. The vasoformative nature is often unclear. In half of cases, a prominent inflammatory infiltrate, often rich in neutrophils, is observed. Nuclear atypia, when present, is mild. Mitotic figures may be present. Intratumoral foci of necrosis may be detected. At the periphery, margins appear infiltrative, in the absence of a fibrous capsule (Fig. 2.58a, b).

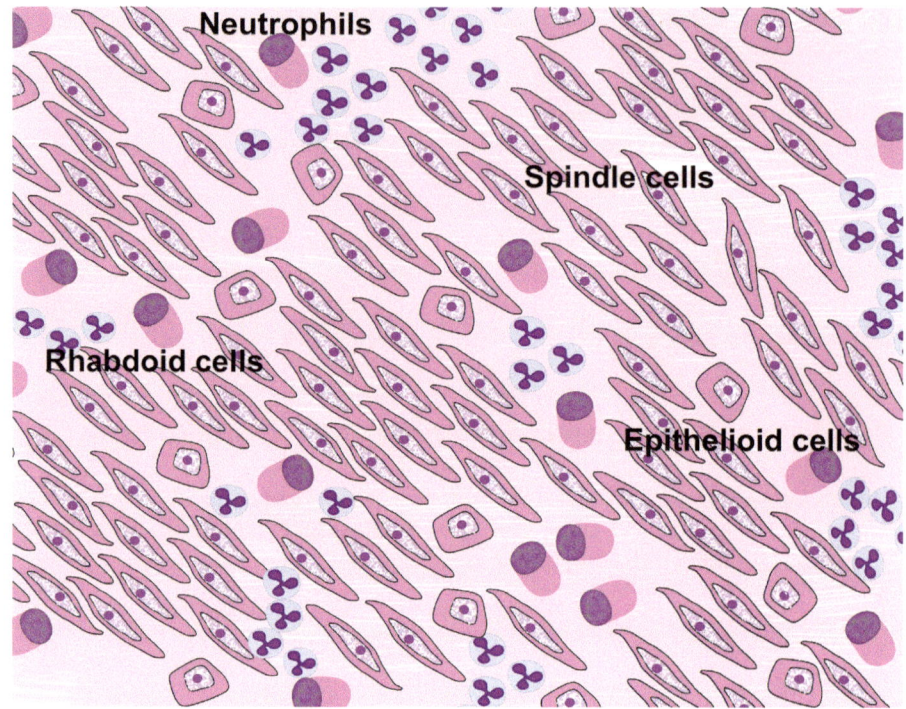

Fig. 2.57 Schematic representation of pseudomyogenic hemangioendothelioma

Immunohistochemistry A strong and diffuse cytoplasmic expression of keratin and nuclear immunostaining for ERG are characteristic features. Recently, a diffuse nuclear immunoreactivity for FOSB (>50% of cells) has been reported in 96% of cases. CD31 may be negative (50% of cases), whereas CD34 and EMA are always negative. Desmin is negative, whereas alpha-SMA may be focally expressed (Fig. 2.58c, d).

Molecular Genetics A translocation between chromosomes 7 and 19 has been reported in a subset of tumors, involving a *SERPINE1-FOSB* fusion.

Prognosis Recurrences and/or appearance of new nodules in the same region are reported in 60% of patients. Metastases are rare, but they may occur many years after the clinical presentation of the disease.

Differential Diagnosis *(1) Epithelioid sarcoma (ES):* ES lacks the fascicles, the sheet arrangement of tumor cells, and the myoid-like spindle cells. ES shows immunoreactivity for EMA and often for CD34, but most importantly the loss of INI1, which is maintained in PHE. *(2) Epithelioid hemangioendothelioma (EHE):*

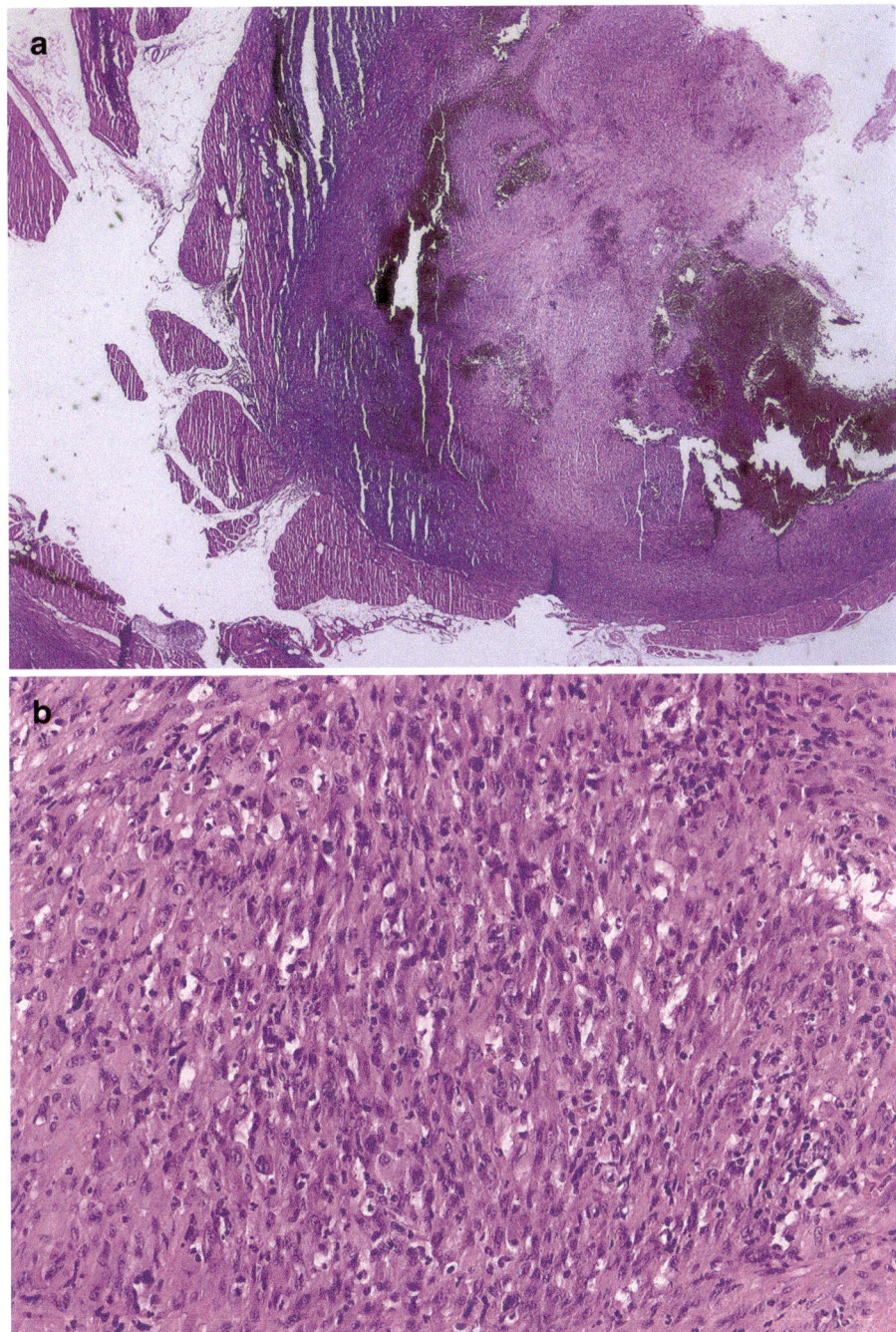

Fig. 2.58 Pseudomyogenic hemangioendothelioma in an 18-year-old male with lesions in leg and arm at low- (**a**) and high-power field (**b**) (HE-stained section), showing the spindled to epithelioid character; immunohistochemistry for keratins at low- (**c**) and high-power fields (**d**)

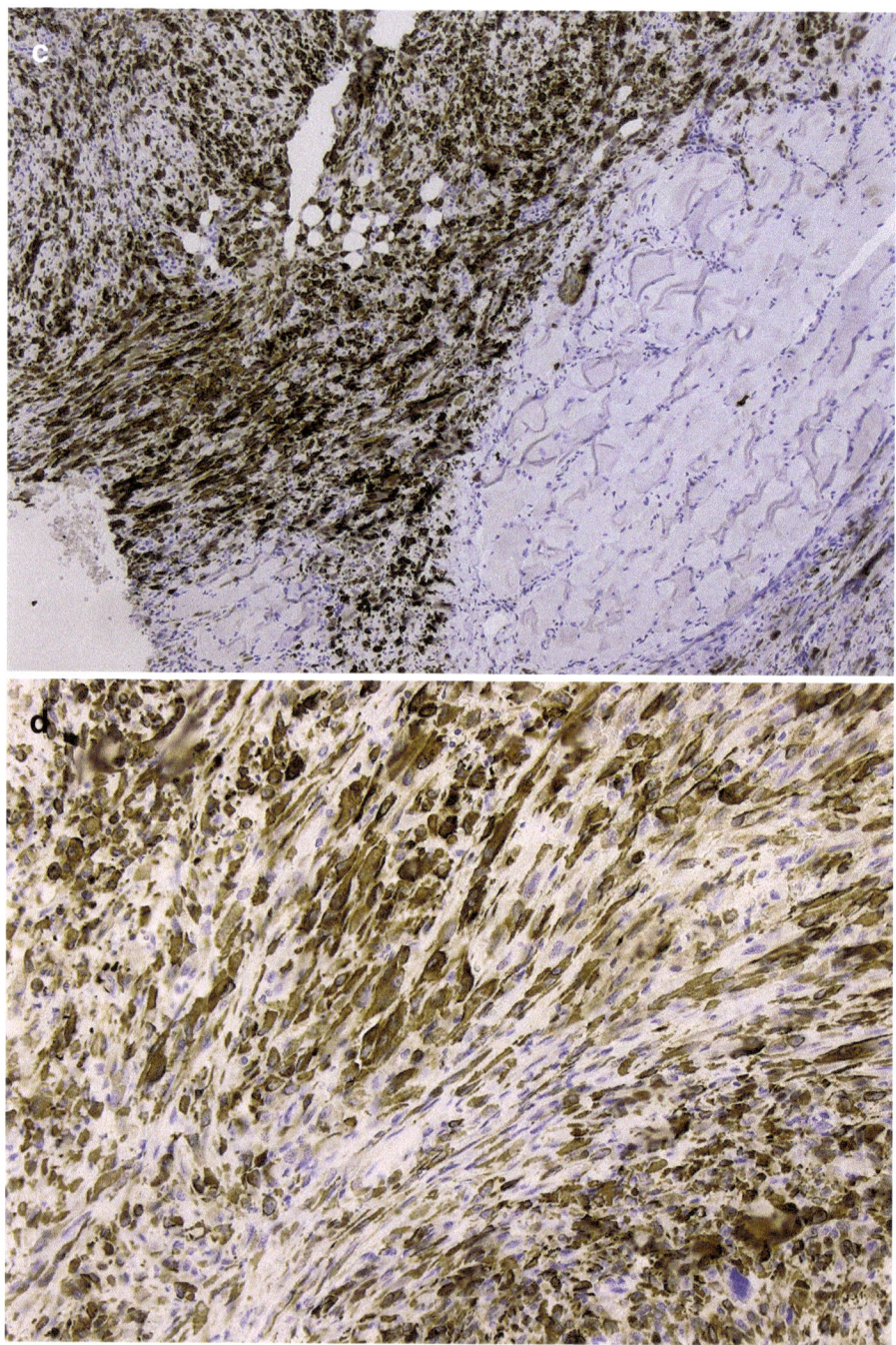

Fig. 2.58 (continued)

epithelioid tumor cells are arranged in cords surrounded by a myxohyaline stroma. EHE is characterized by the expression of CD31, whereas keratin expression is generally focal and not so strong. *(3) Epithelioid angiosarcoma:* tumor cells are large, with abundant eosinophilic cytoplasm, organized in solid sheets, surrounded by stromal hemorrhages. Nuclear atypia is high. *(4) Skeletal muscle tumors:* the expression of desmin and myogenin that characterize these neoplasms is always absent in PHE. *(5) Nodular or proliferative fascitis:* CD31 and ERG are not expressed in myofibroblasts.

Epithelioid Hemangioendothelioma (EHE) (Fig. 2.59)

Definition   High-grade vascular tumor, arising in soft tissues, liver, lung, and bones, characterized by a lack of vasoformative character of epithelioid tumor cells and by a myxohyaline stroma.

Age at Presentation   Adults, median age 50.

Gender   No sex predilection.

Localization   Extremites > head and neck > trunk > mediastinum. Deep soft tissues > superficial. Bones, liver, lungs may be affected.

Clinical Course   Highly variable, ranging from indolent to very aggressive forms.

Macroscopy   Solitary deep-sited nodule, not rarely developing around a large vein.

Histology   Infiltrative margins. Cords of large epithelioid cells, with eosinophilic cytoplasm, surrounded by abundant myxohyaline bluish stroma. Nuclei are bland, roundish, centrally located, with small eosinophilic nucleoli. Cytoplasm may be abundant and glassy. The only histological sign of abortive vascular differentiation is represented by cytoplasmic vacuolation that gives rise to the "blister cells." Mitoses are scarce. Intratumoral necrosis absent. Atypia is mild or absent (Fig. 2.60a, b). A transition to frank epithelioid angiosarcoma can be seen.

Immunohistochemistry   Tumor cells express CD31 (Fig. 2.60c) and ERG (Fig. 2.60d). D240 is occasionally expressed. CD34 mainly highlights the contour of cytoplasmic vacuoles of blister cells. Keratin expression may be found. No alpha-SMA positive cuffing. CAMTA1 expression is often present.

Molecular Genetics   T(1;3) (p36;q25), resulting in the *WWTR1-CAMTA1* gene fusion and CAMTA1 expression. A subset shows *TFE3* rearrangement (t(7;19)), with a *YAP1-TFE3* fusion. These tumors show distinct vasoformative features and more voluminous eosinophilic cytoplasm. Nuclear TFE3 expression is present.

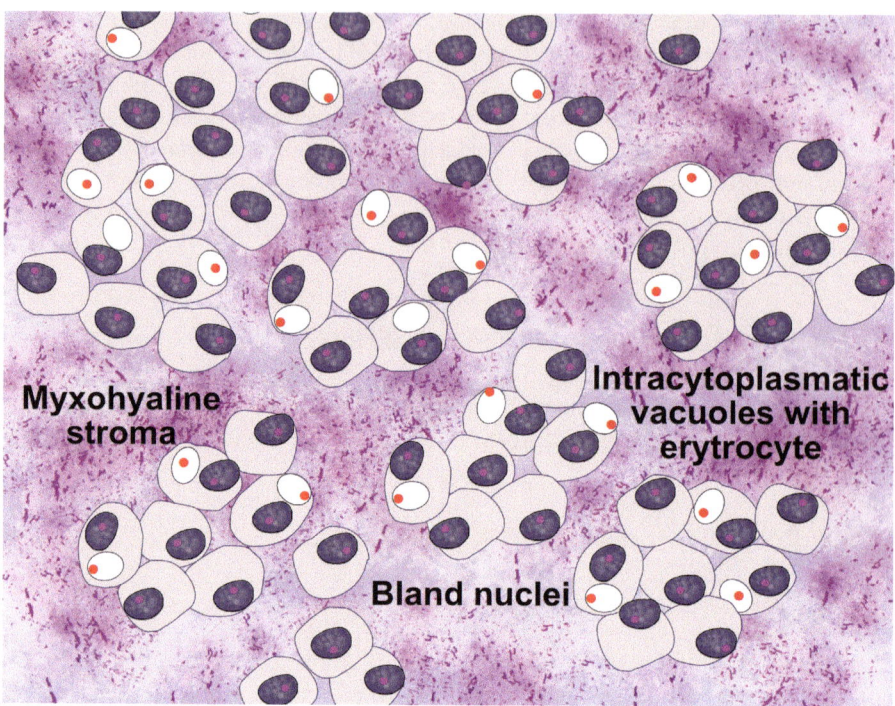

Fig. 2.59 Schematic representation of epithelioid hemangioendothelioma (EHE)

Prognosis Highly variable, mainly depending on tumor size and mitotic index. Tumors of >3 cm in diameter and with >3 mitoses/50 hpf are considered high risk. Wide surgical excision and regional lymph node dissection are the treatment of choice.

Differential Diagnosis *(1) Carcinoma:* strong reactivity for keratin and negativity for vascular markers*; (2) Melanoma:* melanoma markers in the absence of vascular markers*; (3) Malignant mesothelioma:* mesothelioma markers in the absence of vascular markers*; (4) EH*: it shows vascular differentiation*; (5) EAN:* it is localized in the skin, superficial, and shows vascular differentiation*; (6) Myoepithelioma:* it may share with EHE a myxoid stroma and the epithelioid morphology of tumor cells. Immunoreactivity for EMA, CKs, S-100 protein, and GFAP, associated with the negativity of endothelial markers, allow the distinction.

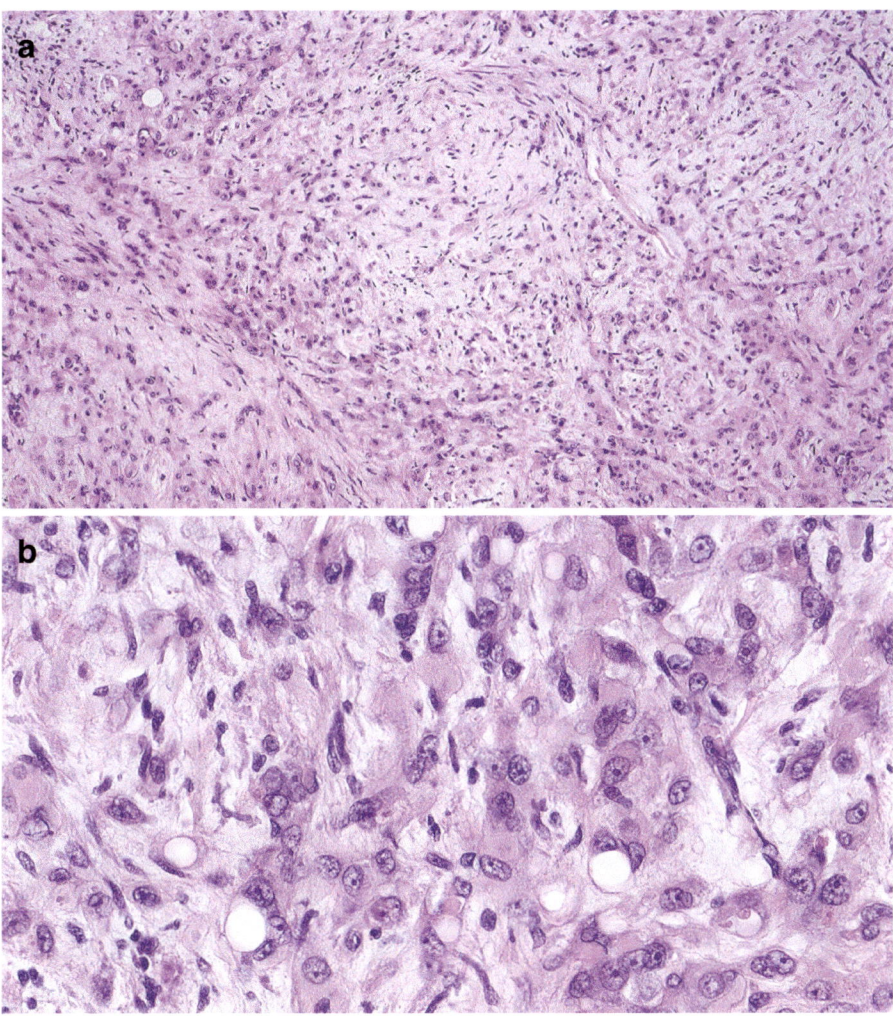

Fig. 2.60 Epithelioid hemangioendothelioma (EHE) from a tumor in the groin of a 27-year-old male at low- (**a**) and high-power fields (**b**) (HE-stained section); immunohistochemistry for CD31 (**c**) and ERG (**d**). Note myxohyaline stroma, the epithelioid cells and the intracytoplasmic vacuoles

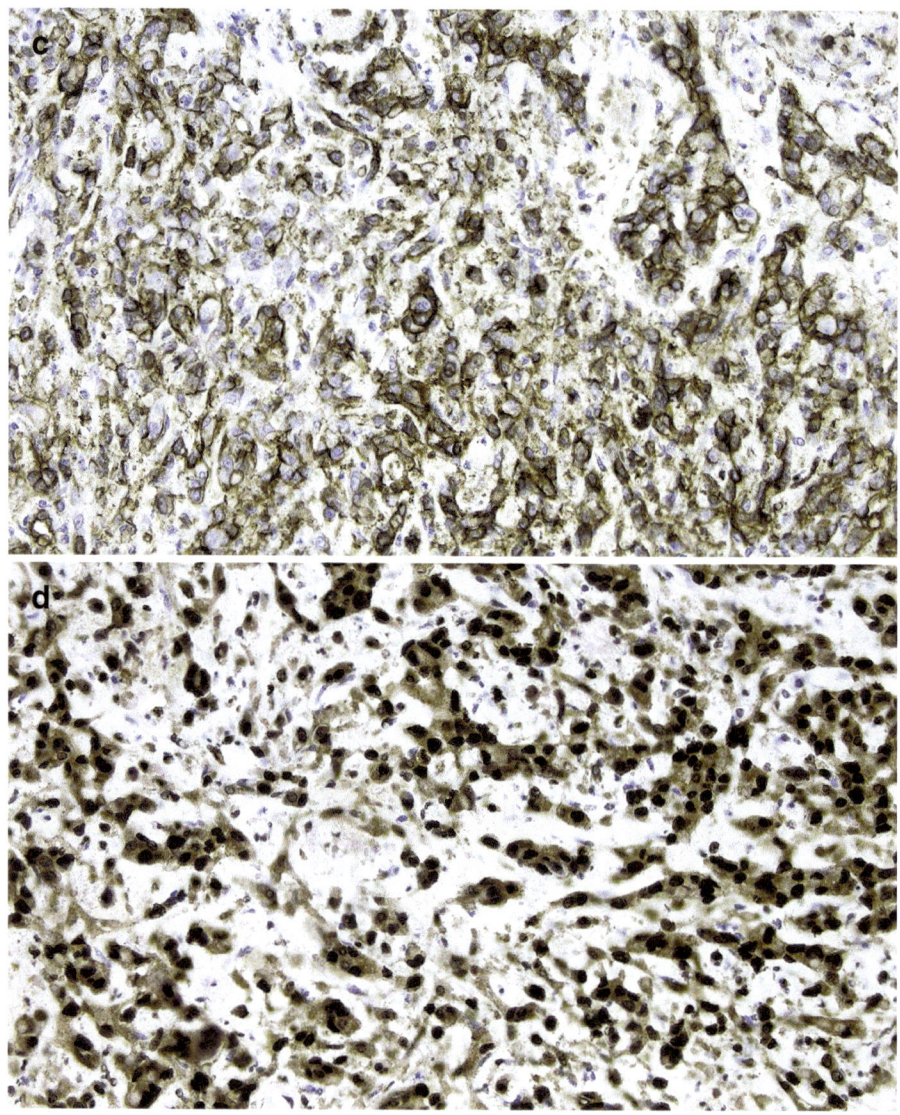

Fig. 2.60 (continued)

Epithelioid Angiosarcoma (EAS) (Fig. 2.61)

Definition Rare malignant vascular neoplasm characterized by the predominance of epithelioid features.

Age at Presentation Adults, middle-aged to elderly.

Gender Predominance of males.

Localization Deep soft tissues of lower extremities (thigh) > retroperitoneum > abdominal cavity > adrenal glands > thyroid gland. Rare in the bone, skin, and mammary glands.

Clinical Course Presenting symptoms: hematoma in deep soft tissues, enteral bleeding, anemia, hemoperitoneum, hemothorax.

Macroscopy Hemorrhagic mass with necrotic areas.

Histology Lobular or nodular growth pattern. Infiltrative margins. Large epithelioid cells, with abundant glassy cytoplasm and large vesicular nuclei, are mainly arranged in solid nests and sheets. Nucleoli are often prominent, scattered cytoplasmic vacuoles may be detected. Mitoses are frequent. Tumor cells may be separated by slit-like spaces, collagenous stroma, or extravasated red blood cells. Pseudo-glandular or pseudopapillary structures are focally found. Intratumoral necrosis and hemorrhages are frequently found. A lympho-plasmocytic infiltrate, with scattered neutrophils, may be present. At the periphery, a vasoformative character may be found, with dilated tumor vessels lined by atypical endothelial cells (Fig. 2.62a, b).

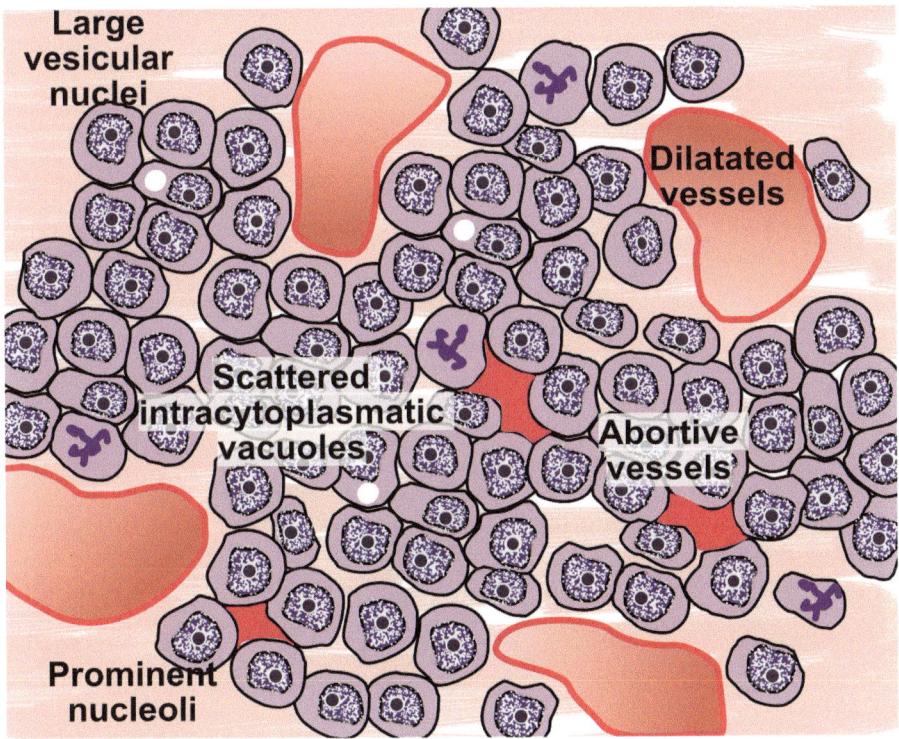

Fig. 2.61 Schematic representation of epithelioid angiosarcoma (EAS)

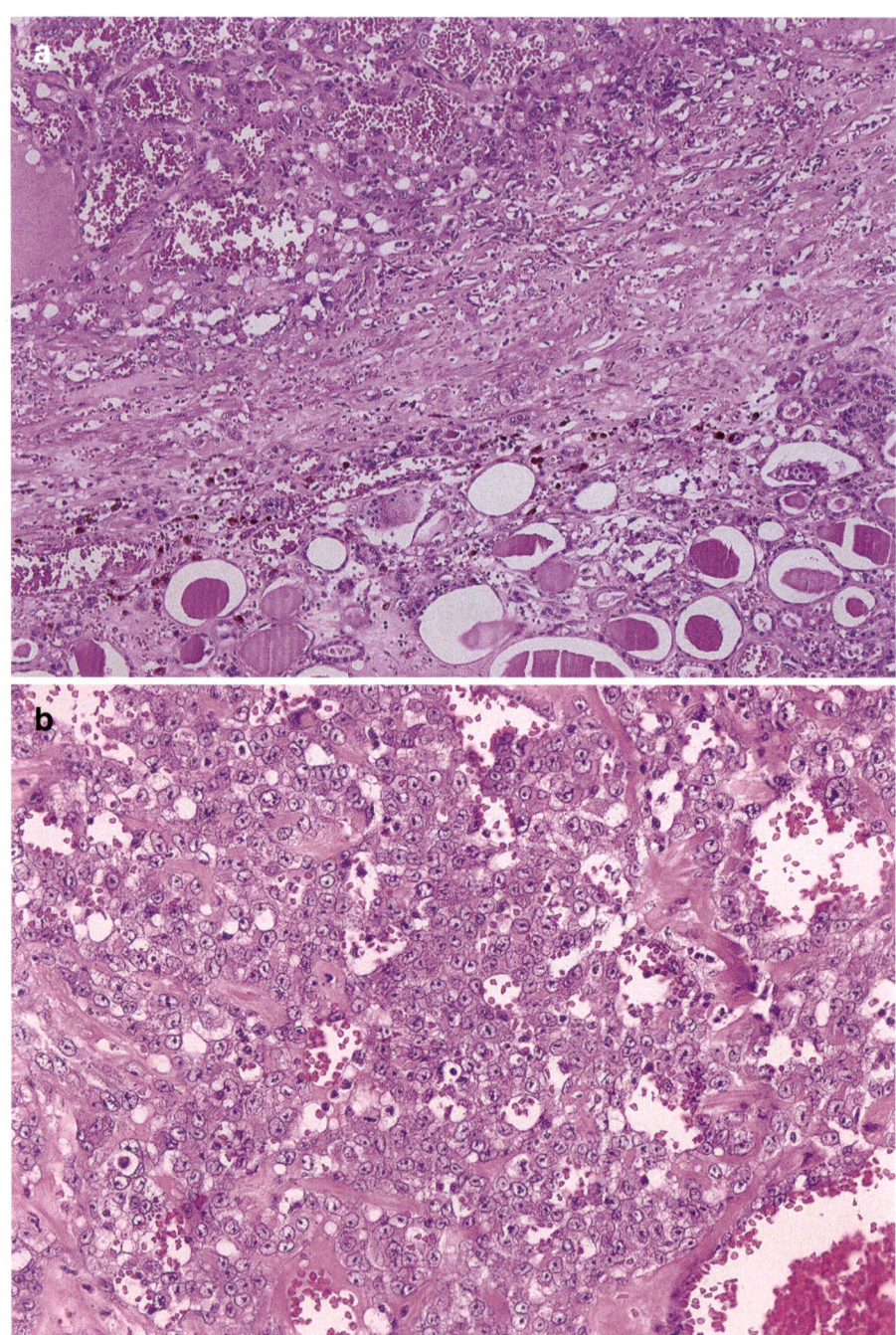

Fig. 2.62 Epithelioid angiosarcoma (EAS) presenting as thyroid enlargement in a 94-year-old male at low- (a) and high-power fields (b) (HE-stained section); immunohistochemistry for CD31 (c) and keratin (d)

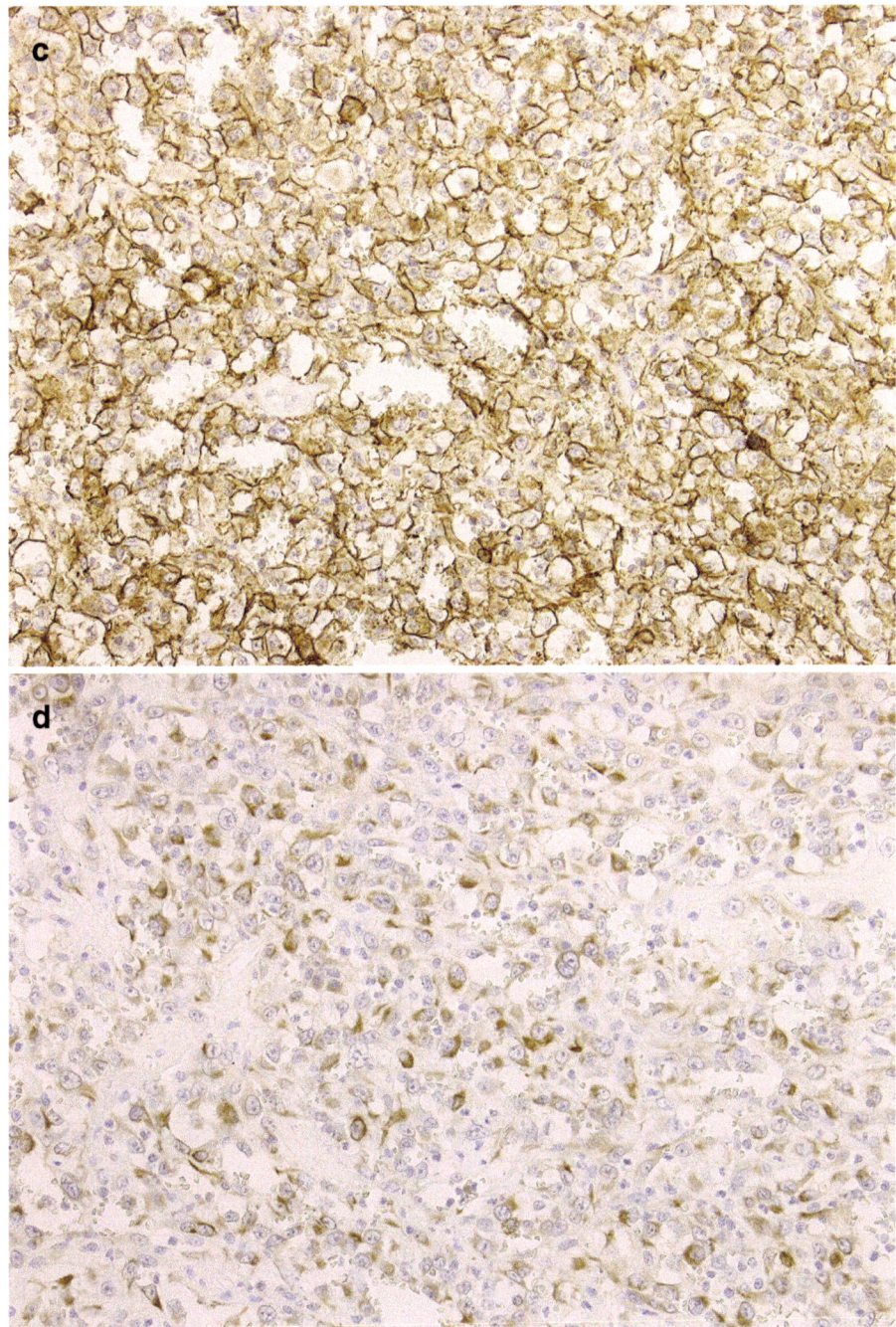

Fig. 2.62 (continued)

Immunohistochemistry CD31 (Fig. 2.62c) and ERG are strongly and diffusely expressed by epithelioid cells. CD34 and D2-40 may be positive. Keratins are expressed in about half of cases (Fig. 2.62d). INI1 expression is maintained.

Molecular Genetics Multiple inconsistent aberrations have been described (*MYC* amplification, *CIC* abnormalities, and *PTRBB* and *PLCG1* mutations).

Prognosis Aggressive soft tissue tumor. Distant metastases occur in more than 50% of patients. High mortality rate.

Differential Diagnosis *(1) EH:* it is a superficial vasoformative lesion, without the anaplastic features of angiosarcoma. *(2) EAN:* superficial lesion, absence of necrosis or atypia, rare mitoses. *(3) EHE:* tumor cells arranged in cords set in a myxohyaline stroma, no/minimal atypia. *(4) Epithelioid sarcoma:* tumor cells express EMA and are negative for INI1. CD31 is negative but ERG can be positive. *(5) Epithelioid MPNST:* tumor cells show strong reactivity for S100 protein. ERG and CD31 are negative. INI1 may be lost (50% of cases).

Tricks for a Correct Diagnosis of Vascular Tumors

1. Benign lesions are much more numerous than malignant ones.
2. Multifocal presentation does not always equal metastatic disease and aggressive behavior (see spindle cell/epithelioid hemangioma, kaposiform/pseudomyogenic hemangioendothelioma).
3. The presence of numerous mitoses and high cellularity is per se not a sign of malignancy. Pediatric benign vascular tumors may show many mitoses.
4. A well-circumscribed, lobular architecture, well-formed vessels with a single layer of endothelial cells surrounded by layer of actin-positive pericytes generally favor a benign lesion.
5. Distinction between malformation and benign neoplasm is often impossible.
6. CD31 is a very sensitive endothelial marker, but it also stains macrophages. It is best to combine CD31 with ERG staining. Nuclear expression of ERG represents a useful tool for defining the vascular nature of a soft tissue tumor. ERG is not restricted to endothelial cells, being expressed in Ewing-like sarcoma, 50% of prostate carcinomas, chloromas, cartilage tumors, and some epithelioid sarcomas.
7. Epithelioid vascular tumors may show reactivity for cytokeratins. The contemporary expression of CD31 and ERG allows a correct diagnosis.
8. Post-radiation angiosarcoma is characterized by strong immunoreactivity and amplification for C-MYC; on the contrary, a radiation-induced atypical vascular lesion is not.

9. Infiltrative margins, a dissecting growth pattern, complex anastomosing channels, endothelial multilayering, and cytological atypia are always worrisome findings.
10. The clinical context is extremely important (age, location, immunosuppression, radiation).
11. HHV8 is a very specific and sensitive marker for Kaposi sarcoma, but the nuclear granular expression may be very faint in early stages.

Essential Bibliography

1. Ko JS, Billings SD. Diagnostically challenging epithelioid vascular tumors. Surg Pathol. 2015;8:331–51.
2. Antonescu CR, Chen HW, Zhang L, et al. ZFP36-FOSB fusion defines a subset of epithelioid hemangioma with atypical features. Genes Chromosom Cancer. 2014;53:951–9.
3. Doyle LA, Fletcher CDM, Hornick JL. Expression of CAMTA1 distinguishes epithelioid hemangioendothelioma from histologic mimics. Am J Surg Pathol. 2016;40:94–102.
4. Hornick JL, Fletcher CDM. Pseudomyogenic hemangioendothelioma: a distinctive often multicentric tumor with indolent behaviour. Am J Surg Pathol. 2011;35:190–201.
5. Hornick JL. In: Leslie KO, Wick MR, editors. Practical soft tissue pathology. A diagnostic approach. Pattern Recognition Series. Philadelphia: Elsevier-Saunders; 2019.
6. Hornick JL. Novel uses of immunohistochemistry in the diagnosis and classification of soft tissue tumors. Modern Pathol. 2014;27:S47–63.
7. Huang SC, Zhang L, Sung YS, et al. Recurrent CIV gene abnormalities in angiosarcomas: a molecular study of 120 cases with concurrent investigation of PLCG1, KDR, MYC and FLT4 gene alterations. Am J Surg Pathol. 2016;40:645–55.
8. McLemore MS, Huo L, Deavers MT. Cutaneous epithelioid angiomatous nodule of the chest wall with expression of estrogen receptor: a mimic of carcinoma and a potential diagnostic pitfall. J Cutan Pathol. 2011;38:818–22.
9. Prenen H, Smeets D, Mazzone M, Lambrechts D, Sagaert X, Sciot R. Phospholipase C gamma 1 (PLCG1) R707Q mutation is counterselected under targeted therapy in a patient with hepatic angiosarcoma. Oncotarget. 2015;6:36418–25.
10. Shustef E, Kazlouskaya V, Prieto VG, Ivan D, Aung PP. Cutaneous angiosarcoma: a current update. J Clin Pathol. 2017;70:917–25.
11. Shon W, Billings SD. Cutaneous malignant vascular neoplasms. Clin Lab Med. 2017;37:633–46.
12. Antonescu C. Malignant vascular tumors – an update. Mod Pathol. 2014;27:S30–8.
13. Weiss SW, Enzinger FM. Epithelioid hemangioendothelioma: a vascular tumor often mistaken for a carcinoma. Cancer. 1982;50:970–81.
14. WHO Classification of Tumours Editorial Board. Soft tissue and bone tumors. Lyon: IARC Press; 2020.
15. Schaefer IM, CDM F. Recent advances in the diagnosis of soft tissue tumours. Pathology. 2018;50(1):37–48.
16. Antonescu CR, Le Loarer F, Mosquera JM, et al. Novel YAP1-TFE3 fusion defines a distinct subset of epithelioid hemangioendothelioma. Genes Chromosem Cancer. 2013;52:775–84.
17. Folpe AL, Chand EM, Goldblum JR, et al. Expression of Fli-1, a nuclear transcription factor, distinguishes vascular neoplasms from potential mimics. Am J Surg Pathol. 2001;25:1061–6.
18. Miettinen M, Wang ZF, Paetau A, et al. ERG transcription facto ras an immunohistochemical marker for vascular endothelial tumors and prostatic carcinoma. Am J Surg Pathol. 2011;35:432–41.

19. Fernandez AP, Sun Y, Tubbs RR, et al. FISH for MYC amplification and anti-MYC immu-
    nohistochemistry: useful diagnostic tools in the assessment of secondary angiosarcoma and
    atypical vascular proliferations. J Cutan Pathol. 2012;39:234–42.
20. Faa G, Sciot R. Soft Tissue Tumors occurring in the perinatal/infancy setting: 2nd part. J
    Pediatr Neonatal Individ Med. 2018;7(1):e70115.
21. Goldblum JR, Folpe AL, Weiss SW. Enzinger & Weiss's soft tissue tumors. 7th ed. Philadelphia:
    Elsevier; 2020.

Skeletal Muscle Tumors

3

Raf Sciot, Clara Gerosa, Daniela Fanni, Carlo Della Rocca,
Maria Debiec-Rychter, and Gavino Faa

Introduction

As opposed to the general rule that benign soft tissue tumors outnumber the malignant ones, rhabdomyomas are much less frequent than rhabdomyosarcomas (RMS). Skeletal muscle tumors tend to recapitulate different stages of development of skeletal muscle fibers. The prototype immature cell is the rhabdomyoblast, a polygonal cell with copious eccentric eosinophilic cytoplasm. The finding of rhabdomyoblasts is not entirely specific for skeletal muscle tumors and, on its own, will not help to discriminate between benign and malignant. The clinical setting as well as architectural patterns, the presence/absence of atypia, pleomorphism, mitoses and necrosis, are very important in this respect. Rhabdomyoblasts can also be mimicked by "rhabdoid cells," which also have an eccentric eosinophilic cytoplasm but have nothing to do with skeletal muscle differentiation. Thus, immunohistochemical markers like myogenin are of utmost importance in the (differential) diagnosis. It is also clear that the genetic background can be crucial to differentiate between entities and often also to define the prognosis. As such, the fusion-positive infantile spindle cell RMS have a very good prognosis. Embryonal and spindle cell/

R. Sciot
Department of Pathology, KU Leuven, UZ Gasthuisberg, Leuven, Belgium

C. Gerosa · D. Fanni (✉) · G. Faa
Divisione di Anatomia Patologica, Dipartimento di Scienze Mediche e Sanità Pubblica, Università degli Studi di Cagliari, Azienda Ospedaliero-Universitaria di Cagliari, Cagliari, Italy

C. D. Rocca
Dipartimento di Scienze e Biotecnologie Medico-Chirurgiche, Policlinico Umberto I, Rome, Italy

M. Debiec-Rychter
Department of Human Genetics, KU Leuven, UZ Gasthuisberg, Leuven, Belgium

© Springer Nature Switzerland AG 2020
R. Sciot et al. (eds.), *Adipocytic, Vascular and Skeletal Muscle Tumors*, Current Clinical Pathology, https://doi.org/10.1007/978-3-030-37460-0_3

sclerosing RMS lacking genetic abnormalities have a good prognosis and the alveolar, *MYOD1*-mutant spindle cell/sclerosing and pleomorphic RMS have a poor prognosis.

Rhabdomyoma

Definition Rhabdomyoma is a benign neoplasm originating from striated muscle cells. According to its localization, it is subdivided into a cardiac and an extracardiac form. Extracardiac rhabdomyoma may be subdivided into three clinicopathological subtypes: i) adult, ii) fetal (juvenile), and iii) genital rhabdomyoma.

Adult-Type Rhabdomyoma (Fig. 3.1)

Age at Presentation Adult and elderly subjects (> 40 years, mean age 60 years).

Gender Male predominance (M:F = 3:1).

Localization Head and neck: soft tissues, oral cavity, tongue, pharynx, larynx.

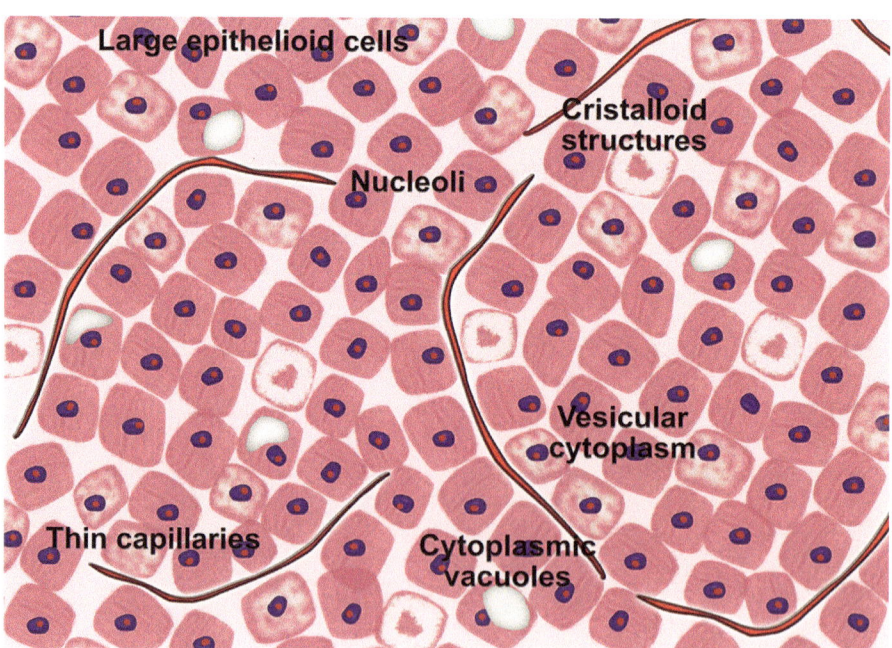

Fig. 3.1 Schematic representation of adult-type rhabdomyoma: large polygonal cells with abundant eosinophilic to vacuolated cytoplasm and a thin capillary network

Clinical Course It generally presents as a single, well-demarcated nodule. Multiple nodules are present in 2–3 out of 10 patients.

Macroscopy Nodule, mean diameter of 3 cm, occasionally polypoid.

Microscopy Adult rhabdomyoma is characterized by round to polygonal, uniform, large epithelioid cells, with abundant eosinophilic cytoplasm, and central small nuclei, occasionally vesicular, with evident nucleoli. Cytoplasmic vacuoles are often found. Thin capillaries, often containing red blood cells, are contained in a delicate stroma encircling tumor cells. Inside the cytoplasm, crystalloid structures may be detected. Very rare mitoses, but no intratumoral necrosis, are seen (Fig. 3.2a).

Variants (1) *The clear cell variant* is characterized by tumor cells with abundant cytoplasmic vacuoles, resulting in a clear cell appearance; (2) *The spider cell variant* is characterized by the finding of tumor cells with delicate cytoplasmic strands emerging from the cell membrane.

Immunohistochemistry Tumor cells are immunoreactive for desmin (Fig. 3.2b), muscle-specific actin (HHF35), and myogenin (Myf4). Smooth muscle actin and S-100 protein may be focally expressed.

Molecular Genetics No specific molecular changes reported.

Prognosis Benign lesion. Complete excision is curative. Recurrences are due to incomplete surgical excision.

Differential Diagnosis (1) *Granular cell tumor:* strong and diffuse immunostaining for S100 protein and CD68; (2) *Hibernoma*: it is characterized by vacuolated brown fat cells; (3) *Crystal-storing histiocytosis*: histiocytes that phagocytosed crystalloid immunoglobulins, in the setting of a lymphoplasmocytic lymphoma, are immunoreactive for CD68 and CD163; (4) *Well-differentiated embryonal rhabdomyosarcoma*: certainly after chemotherapy, this tumor may show a rhabdomyoma-like appearance. The presence of focal nuclear polymorphism and atypia may help in the differential diagnosis, as the clinical history does; (5) *Alveolar soft part sarcoma*: the alveolar growth pattern is usually very prominent, as well as prominent vascular invasion. Desmin expression can be seen in the large polygonal cells, but TFE3 expression is typical and is not present in rhabdomyoma.

Fetal (Juvenile) Rhabdomyoma (Fig. 3.3)

Definition Fetal rhabdomyoma (FRM) is a rare soft tissue tumor of newborns and infants, with a peculiar localization in the head and neck region.

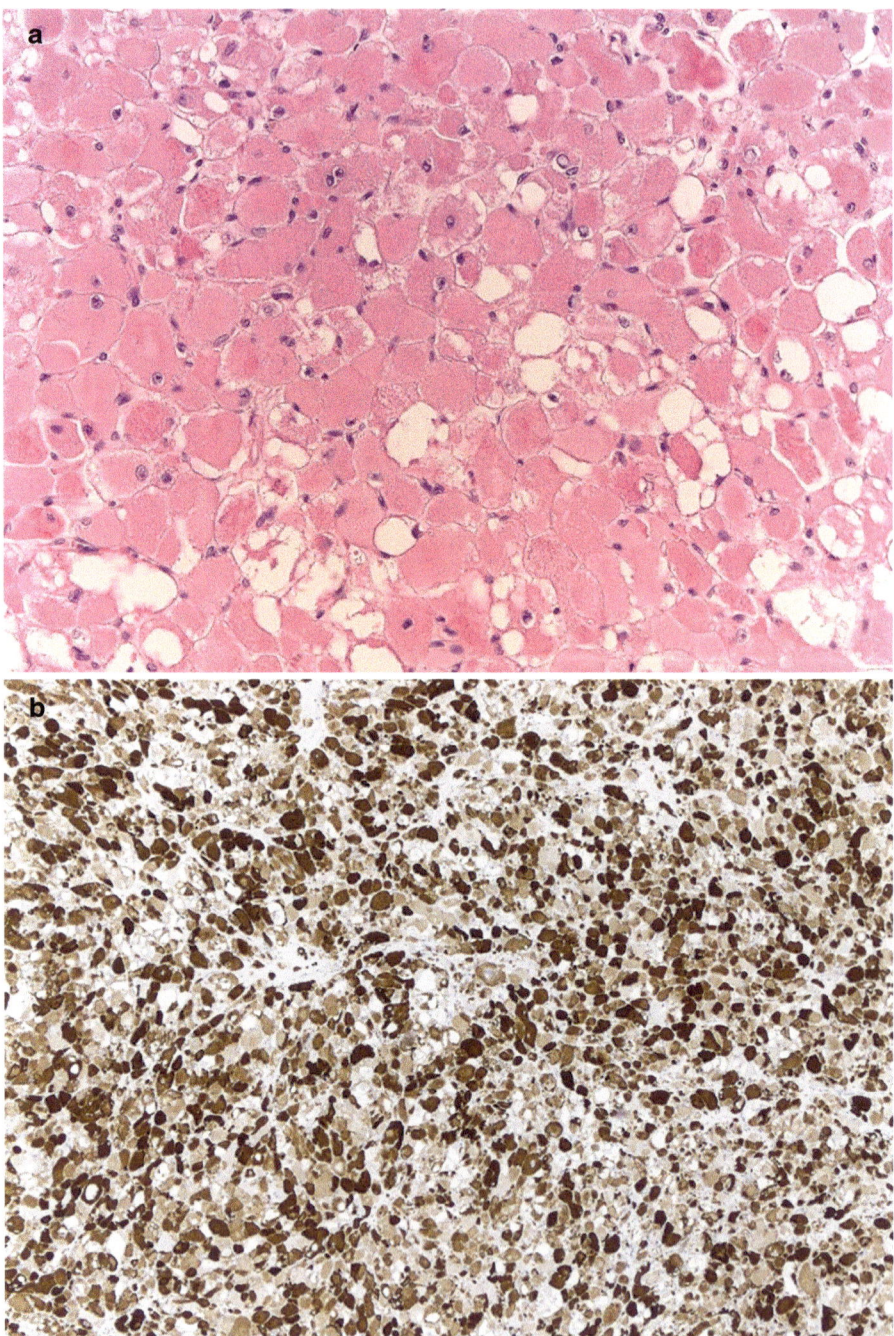

Fig. 3.2 (**a**) Adult-type rhabdomyoma characterized by uniform large epithelioid cells with abundant eosinophilic cytoplasm and central small nuclei, in a 69-year-old female, with a slowly growing mass in the laryngopharynx since about 10 years. (**b**) Desmin positivity in adult-type rhabdomyoma

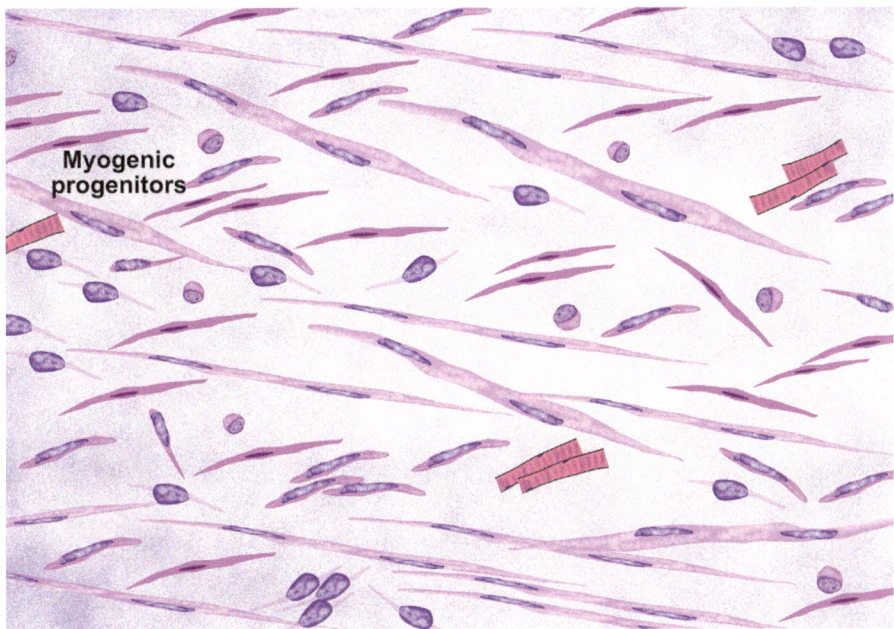

Fig. 3.3 Schematic representation of fetal rhabdomyoma: roundish and spindle cell progenitors in a myxoid stroma with focal mature muscle fibers

Age at Presentation FRM may be congenital, or may present after birth, within the first three years of age. Mean age: 4 years.

Gender Males predominate.

Localization The head and neck are most frequently involved. The trunk, hands, feet, larynx, and the perianal region may also be affected. Rarely, FRM may originate in the tonsil, presenting as a polyp.

Clinical Course Benign lesion. Rare recurrences are due to incomplete excision.

Macroscopy Well-circumscribed mass.

Microscopy The histological picture often recapitulates fetal development of skeletal muscle. Immature spindle mesenchymal progenitor cells, spindle cells with abundant eosinophilic cytoplasm, myotubes, rhabdomyoblasts, myocytes, and muscle cells with evident cross striation may be all observed in variable proportions. Tumor cells are often embedded in a myxoid stroma. The tumor is often well-vascularized, with very prominent thin vessels. No atypia, no intratumoral necrosis, no nuclear polymorphism. Mitoses can be present (Fig. 3.4a, b).

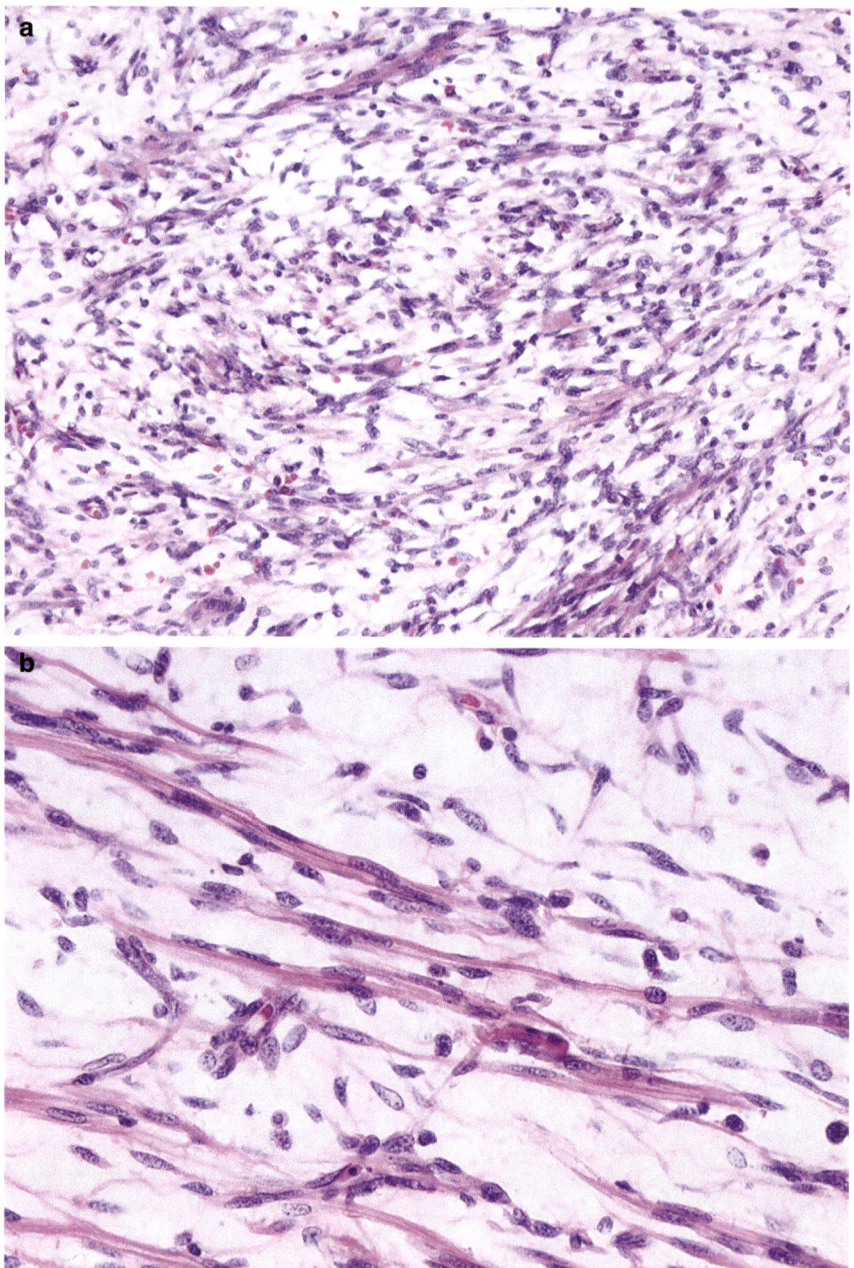

Fig. 3.4 (**a, b**) Fetal rhabdomyoma occurring as a 9 cm subcutaneous mass in the neck of a male newborn, at low power field (**a**) and high power field (**b**), showing immature roundish/spindle mesenchymal progenitor cells, spindle cells, rhabdomyoblasts, myocytes, and muscle cells with evident cross variation in short fascicles, all embedded in a myxoid stroma, (**c**) Desmin expression in fetal rhabdomyoma

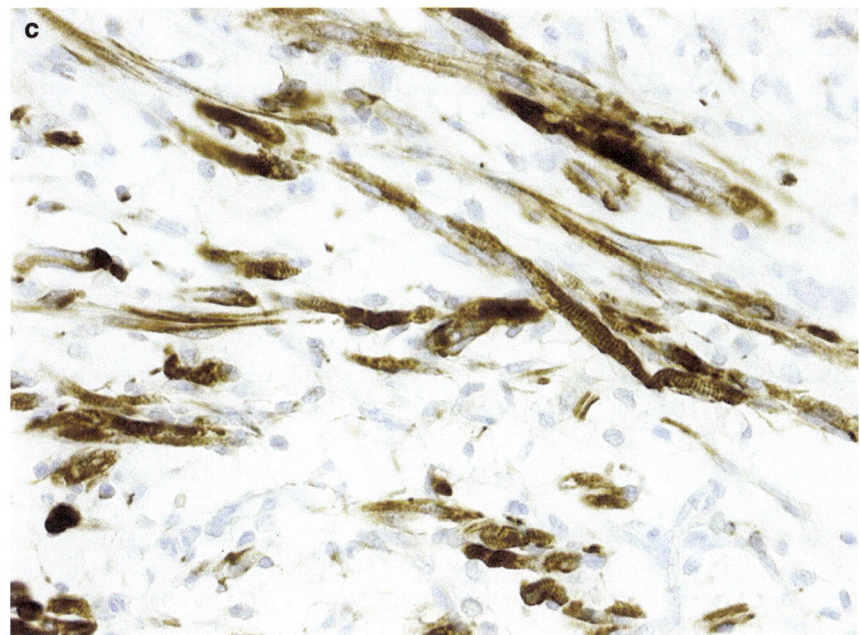

Fig. 3.4 (continued)

Variants (1) Bland immature primitive spindle cells, embedded in a myxoid stroma, characterize the *classical variant*; (2) The *cellular "intermediate" variant* is characterized by a high cellularity, immature spindle cells in fascicles, eosinophilic spindle cells, and scattered rhabdomyoblasts.

Immunohistochemistry Tumor cells are desmin positive (Fig. 3.4c) and diffusely reactive for muscle-specific actin. Scattered myogenin positive differentiated rhabdomyoblasts are often detected.

Molecular Genetics No specific molecular changes. Mutations in the Hedgehog pathway have been occasionally reported.

Prognosis Benign lesion. Complete surgical excision is curative. Local recurrences are uncommon.

Differential Diagnosis (1) *Embryonal or spindle cell rhabdomyosarcoma*: the presence of nuclear atypia and invasion favor the diagnosis of rhabdomyosarcoma.

Genital Rhabdomyoma (Fig. 3.5)

Definition Rare benign tumor, with skeletal muscle differentiation, localized in the genitalia.

Age at Presentation Middle-aged women, mean age 45 years.

Gender Females predominate. Rare cases have been described in males.

Localization Vagina > vulva > cervix. Rarely in the epididymis.

Clinical Course Solitary, nodular, or polypoid submucosal mass. Bleeding may be the presenting symptom.

Macroscopy Nodular or polypoid tumor, well circumscribed (usually <2 cm).

Microscopy A spindle cell proliferation, arranged in fascicles, with abundant eosinophilic cytoplasm and occasional cross striations is seen. Eosinophilic large tumor cells are embedded in a loose fibrous stroma. No mitoses, nor significant atypia (Fig. 3.6).

Immunohistochemistry Tumor cells are immunoreactive for the classical skeletal muscle markers.

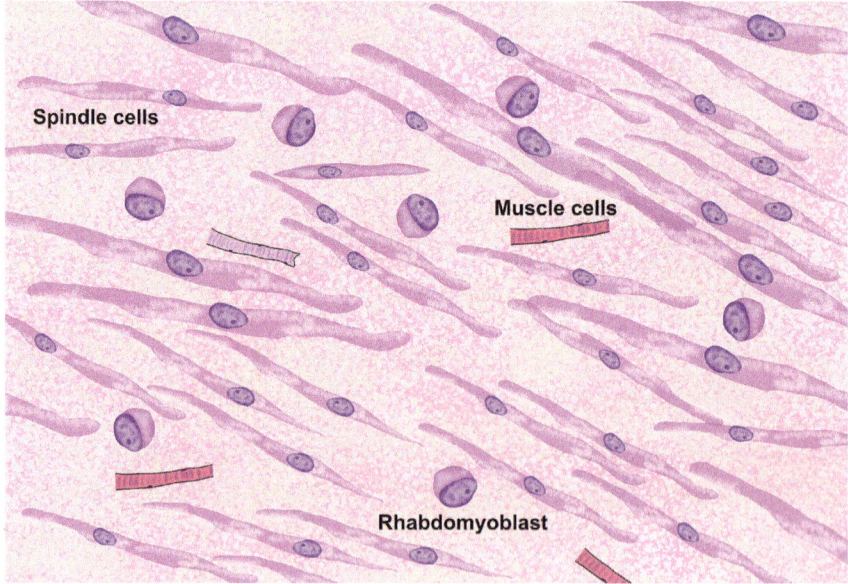

Fig. 3.5 Schematic representation of genital rhabdomyoma: rhabdomyoblasts, immature spindle cells, and mature striated muscle cells

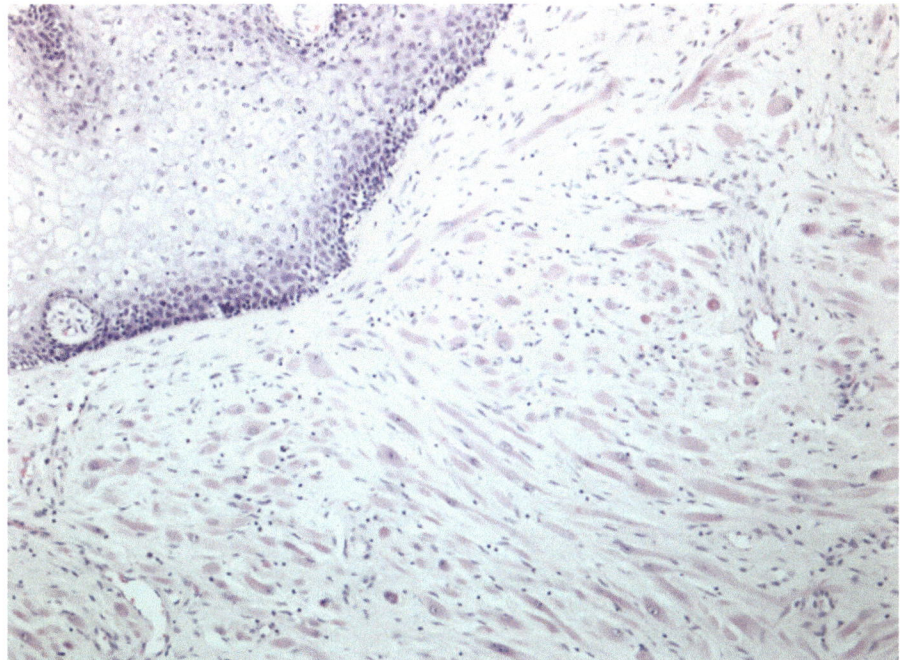

Fig. 3.6 Genital rhabdomyoma, characterized by spindle cells proliferation arranged in short fascicles and eosinophilic large tumor cells embedded in a loose fibrous stroma, from the vagina of a 35-year-old woman

Molecular Genetics No specific changes.

Prognosis Benign lesion, complete excision is curative.

Differential Diagnosis (1) *Embryonal rhabdomyosarcoma*: finding of atypia, frequent mitotic figures, and a cambium layer, associated with lower age at presentation, are in favor of the diagnosis of embryonal rhabdomyosarcoma.

Embryonal Rhabdomyosarcoma (Fig. 3.7)

Definition The most frequent sarcoma in children, and the most frequent subtype of rhabdomyosarcoma, showing embryonic skeletal muscle features.

Age at Presentation Children, 3–12 years.

Gender Slight male predominance.

Localization Head and neck > genitourinary tract > liver > retroperitoneum > nasopharynx > biliary tract.

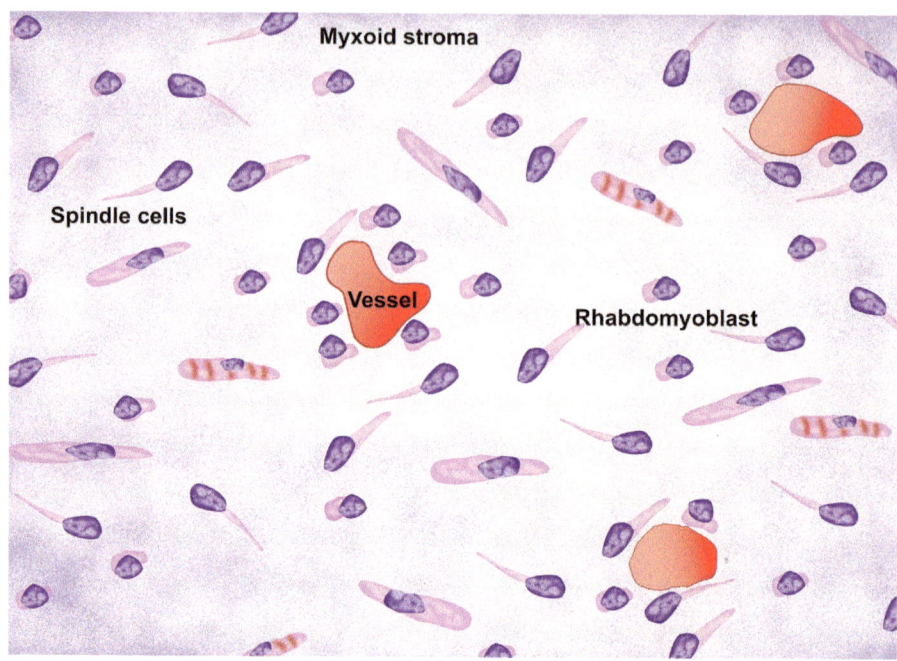

Fig. 3.7 Schematic representation of embryonal RMS: rhabdomyoblasts with large atypical nuclei embedded in a myxoid stroma

Clinical Course Good prognosis, and responsiveness to chemotherapy even in the presence of metastasis.

Macroscopy Ill-defined, friable mass, white in color. In the typical presentation, it appears as a polyp originating beneath the mucosa of the nose, upper respiratory tract, bladder, or vagina.

Microscopy Heterogeneity of tumor cells characterizes this tumor. A mixture of undifferentiated spindle and round cells surrounded by a myxoid stroma, with occasional more differentiated elongated cells with eosinophilic cytoplasma and cross striations, characterizes the conventional variant. Tumor cells show the tendency to aggregate around vascular structures (Fig. 3.8a).

Variants (1) *Botryoid variant*: is characterized by a polypoid, grape-like appearance and by a cambium layer, i.e., the presence of foci of tumor cells densely aggregated beneath the mucosal surface (Fig. 3.8b, c); (2) *Anaplastic variant*: it is characterized by the presence of abundant very atypical tumor cells, atypical mitotic figures, and sometimes by heterologous chondroid differentiation (Fig. 3.8d, e).

Immunohistochemistry Desmin and muscle-specific actin are widely expressed. Immunostaining for myogenin is often focal, being more strong in the nuclei of undifferentiated tumor cells and absent in more differentiated cells. Myogenin expression in embryonal RMS is typically less prominent than in the alveolar subtype.

Molecular Genetics Numerical chromosomal changes and allelic loss of 11p15 are frequent in embryonal RMS. Aberrations of the *RAS/AKT* pathway have been described as well.

Prognosis Prognosis is excellent, with 70% disease-free survival in general. Chemotherapy (often inducing skeletal muscle differentiation (Fig. 3.8f)), surgery, and radiotherapy are involved. The stage (lungs, lymph nodes, liver, brain are the most frequent metastatic sites) and age at diagnosis are most important for prognosis. Children of 1 to 9 years show a better outcome. The type and site are also important. The botryoid variant has the best prognosis and the anaplastic variant the worse. The orbita and the paratesticulum are prognostically the best sites.

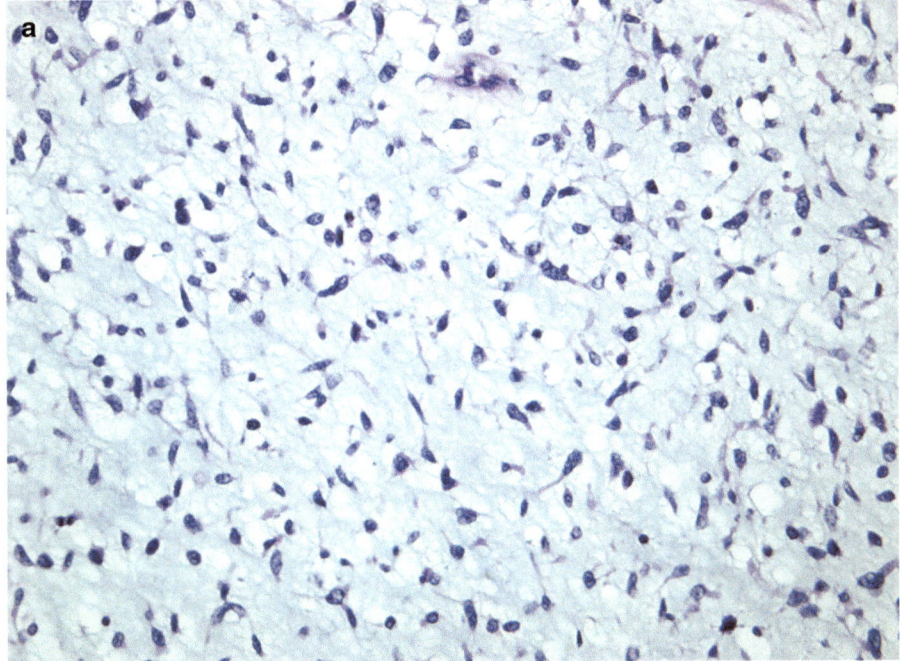

Fig. 3.8 (**a**) Embryonal RMS with a mixture of undifferentiated spindle and round cells surrounded by a myxoid stroma. Note the atypical nuclei. (**b**) Botryoid variant of embryonal RMS: tumor cells are overcrowded beneath the epithelial surface, forming a "cambium" layer, from a cervical polypoid lesion of a 46-year-old female. (**c**) Positive immunohistochemistry for myogenin in the botryoid variant of embryonal RMS. (**d**) Anaplastic variant of embryonal RMS characterized atypical tumor cells and atypical mitotic figures. (**e**) Anaplastic variant of embryonal RMS with chondroid differentiation. (**f**) Embryonal RMs after chemotherapy

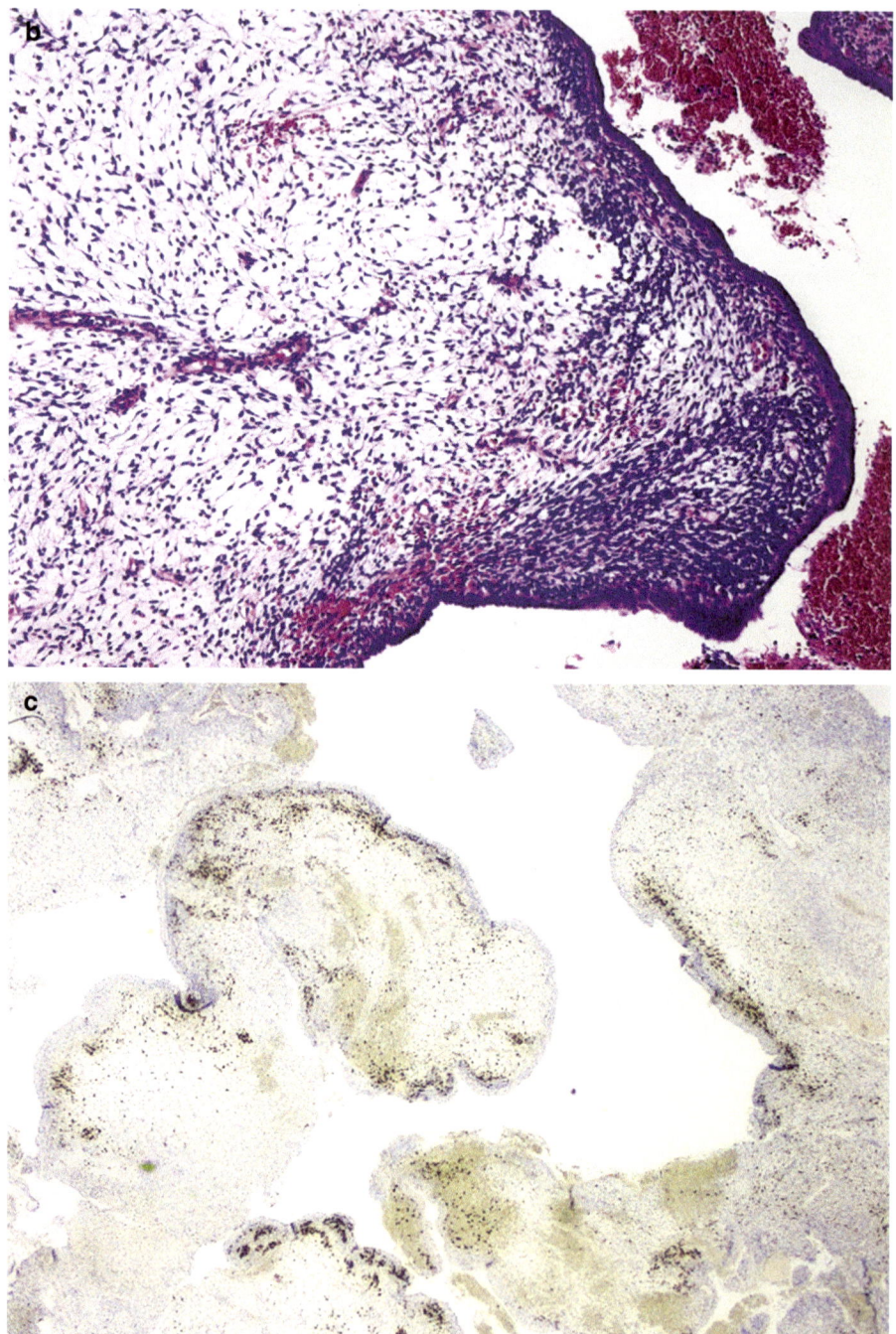

Fig. 3.8 (continued)

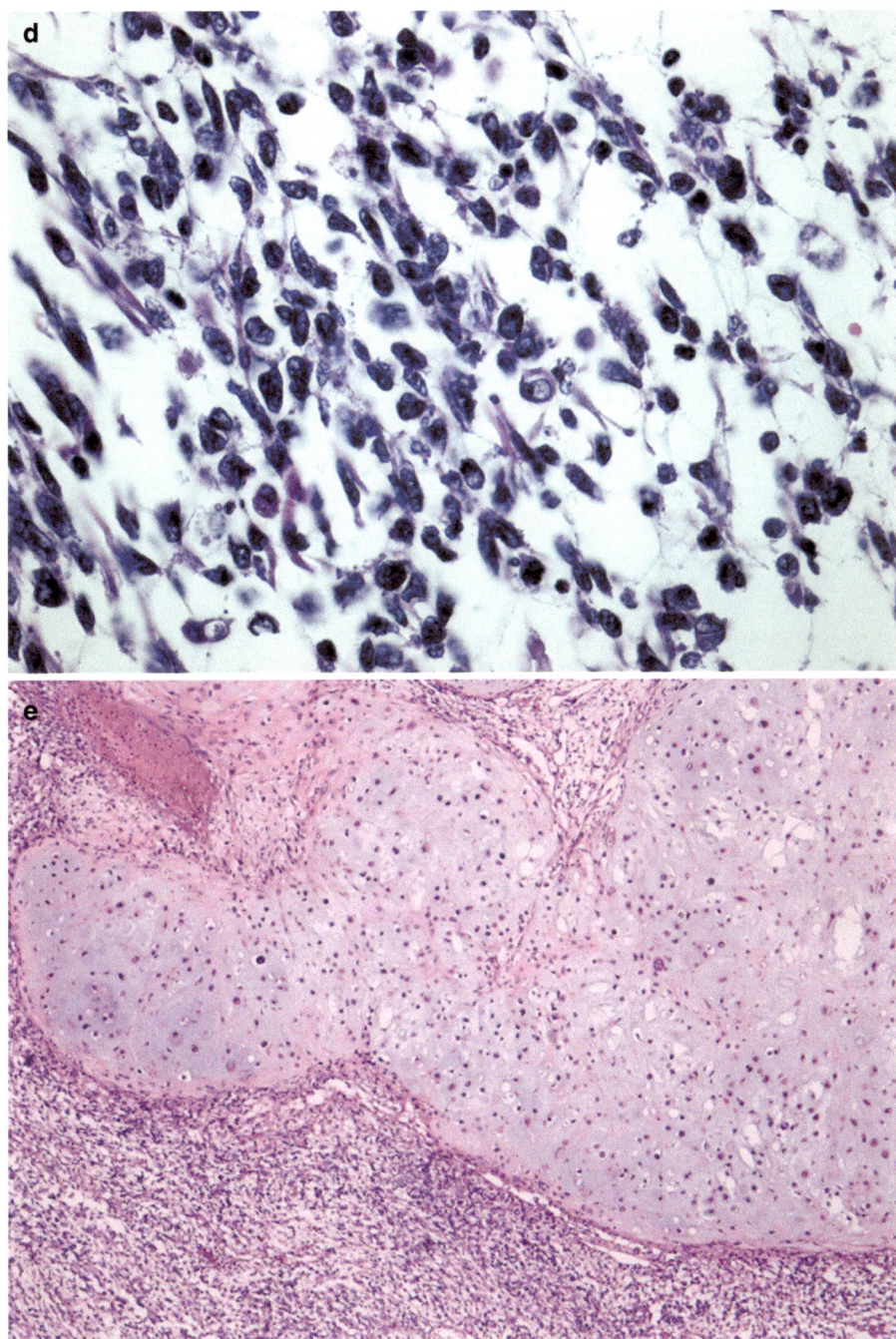

Fig. 3.8 (continued)

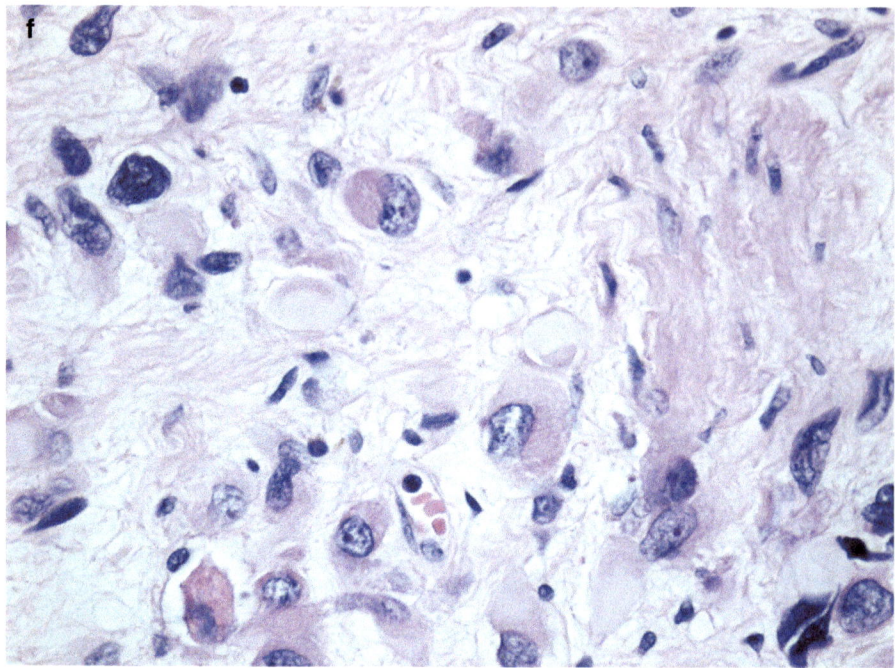

Fig. 3.8 (continued)

Differential Diagnosis (1) *Alveolar rhabdomyosarcoma*, especially the solid variant: cells are generally larger and the nuclear staining for myogenin is typically uniform, strong, and diffuse, contrasting with the focal and heterogeneous immunostaining typical of the embryonal subtype. Molecular genetics show typical changes in the majority of cases.

Alveolar Rhabdomyosarcoma (Fig. 3.9)

Definition It is the second most common (25–30%) rhabdomyosarcoma, presenting in childhood and adolescence.

Age at Presentation The highest incidence is between 10 and 25 years.

Gender No sex predilection.

Localization Extremities (forearm) > head and neck > trunk > pelvis.

Clinical Course Aggressive tumor with poor prognosis, with hematogenic or lymphogenic spread at diagnosis occurring in 25–30% of patients.

Macroscopy A fleshy mass with variable fibrous/hemorrhagic areas.

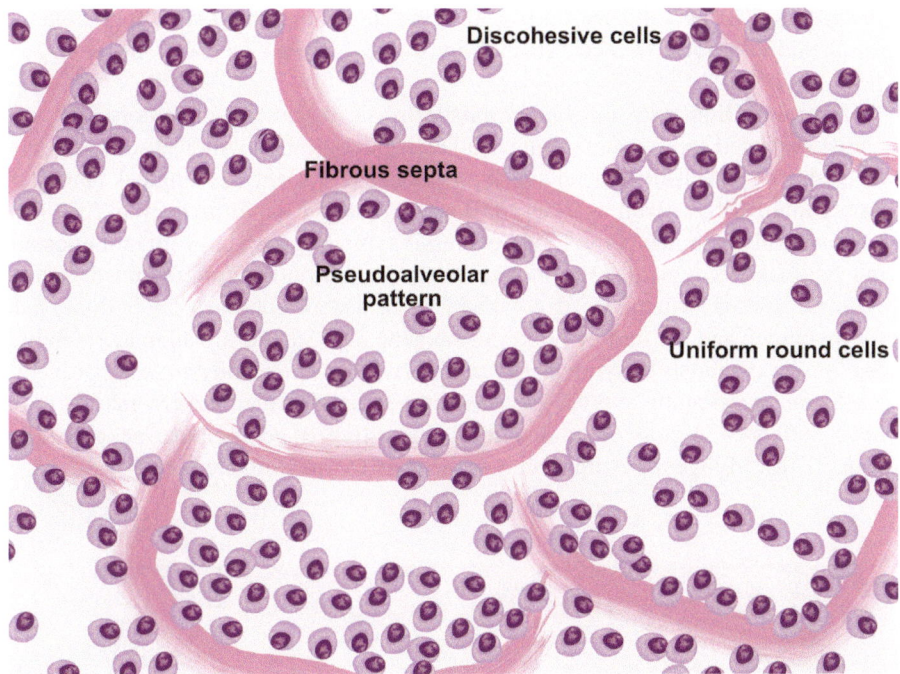

Fig. 3.9 Schematic representation of alveolar RMS: round discohesive cells in pseudoalveolar pattern supported by fibrous septa

Microscopy The typical appearance of the conventional type is that of nests of uniform small round cells separated by fibrous septa, with a discohesive aspect in the center, giving rise to a pseudoalveolar pattern (Fig. 3.10a). In some cases, the tumor cells may show a clear cytoplasm, and the stroma may be very sclerotic.

Variant (1) *Solid variant*: larger tumor cells, with scant cytoplasm (blue tumor), very thin fibrous septa, and frequent giant cells (Fig. 3.10b).

Immunohistochemistry Strong and diffuse nuclear reactivity for myogenin (Fig. 3.10c) and strong cytoplasmic reactivity for desmin. Olig2 may be a new surrogate marker for the *PAX3/7-FOXO1* fusion. ALK expression is often present. Positivity for keratins and neuroendocrine markers can be seen, more often in the head and neck tumors of adults (Fig. 3.10d–h).

Molecular Genetics t(2;13), resulting in fusion of the *PAX3/FOXO1* genes, and t(1;13), resulting in the fusion of the *PAX7/FOXO1* genes, are detected in 85% of patients. *ALK* gene rearrangements are possible, but not therapeutic. About 15% of patients are fusion-negative, or show alternative rare fusions, including *PAX3-NCOA1* or *PAX3-AFX* fusion genes. Recently, distinct methylation profiles have been proposed to differentiate fusion-positive and fusion-negative rhabdomyosarcomas.

Prognosis The overall survival is <50%, the stage being the major predictive factor. In addition, *PAX3-FOXO1* fusions are worse than *PAX7-FOXO1* fusions.

Differential Diagnosis (1) *Embryonal RMS*: heterogeneity of tumor cells, with undifferentiated spindle and small round cells intermingled with well-differentiated cells showing well-developed cross striations, is typical histological marker of embryonal RMS, as well as more focal expression pattern of myogenin. (2) *Ewing sarcoma*: diffuse honeycomb CD99 expression, often associated with immunostaining for FLI1, is typical. (3) *Synovial sarcoma*: the poorly differentiated form of synovial sarcoma can mimic alveolar RMS. The absence of reactivity of tumor cells for myogenin and the finding of the fusion gene *SYT-SSX1/2* are all markers indicative for the diagnosis of synovial sarcoma. (4) *Neuroendocrine carcinoma*: alveolar RMS can occasionally express keratins and neuroendocrine markers, mainly in the head and neck region of adults, thus suggesting a neuroendocrine carcinoma (Fig. 3.10i). Myogenin expression is mandatory to discriminate both.

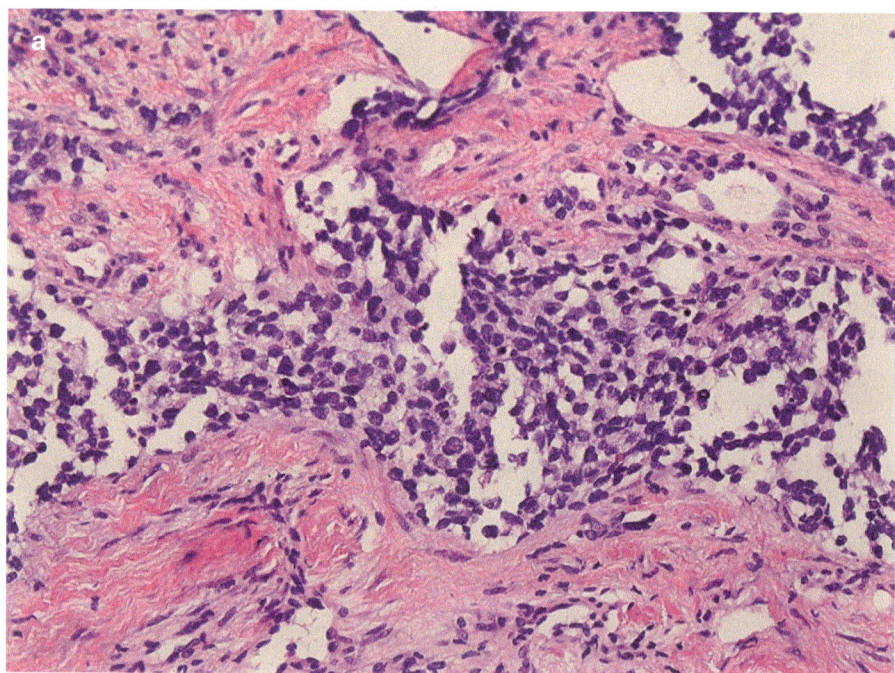

Fig. 3.10 (**a**) Typical appearance of convention alveolar RMS with nests of uniform and small round cells separated by fibrous septa, from a tumor localized in the pelvic floor of a 14-year-old boy. (**b**) Solid variant of alveolar RMS characterized by large tumor cells and thin fibrous septa, from a tumor near the kidney of a 45-year-old male. (**c**) Myogenin positivity in alveolar RMS. (**d**) Solid variant of alveolar RMS in head and neck with neuroendocrine features. This was an unusual clinical and immunohistochemical presentation in a 61-year-old male showing a tumor in the nasopharynx suspicious for a neuroendocrine tumor. (**e**) Absence of keratin expression in the tumor seen in **d**. (**f**) Synaptophysin, (**g**): NCAM (CD56), (**h**): Desmin, and (**i**): Myogenin positivity in the tumor seen in **d**. (**j**): Break-apart *FOXO1*/13q14 (Vysis) FISH in alveolar RMS

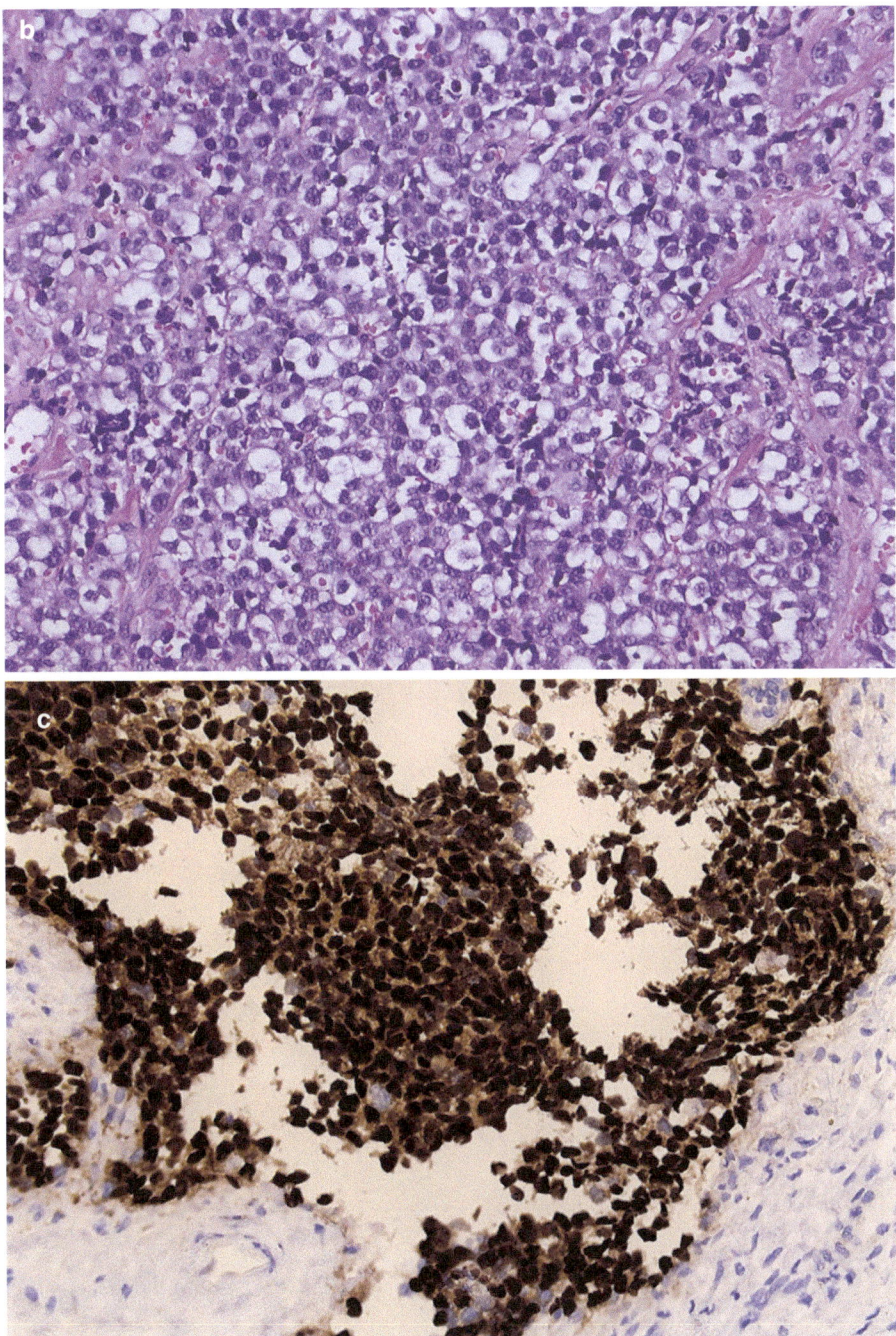

Fig. 3.10 (continued)

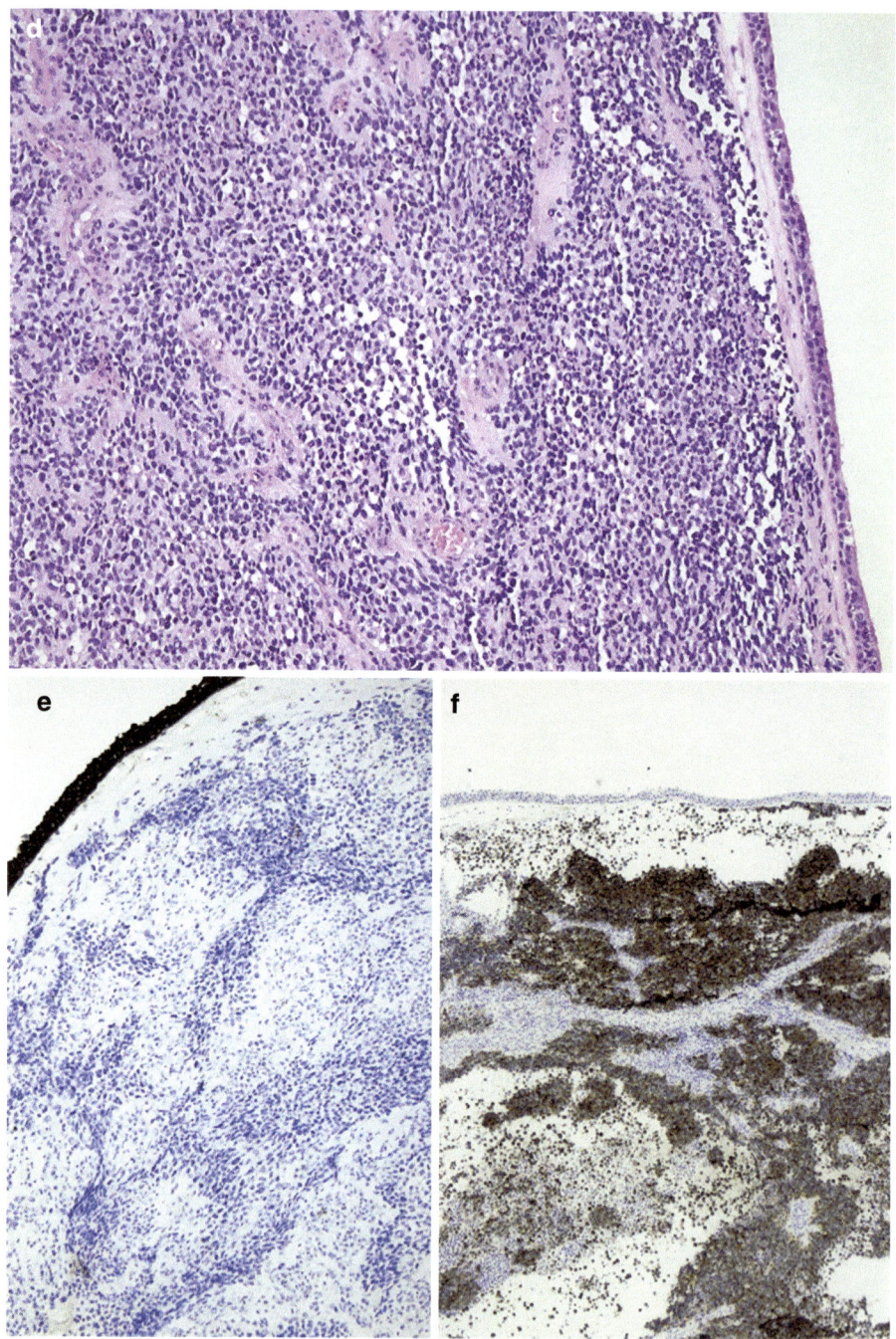

Fig. 3.10 (continued)

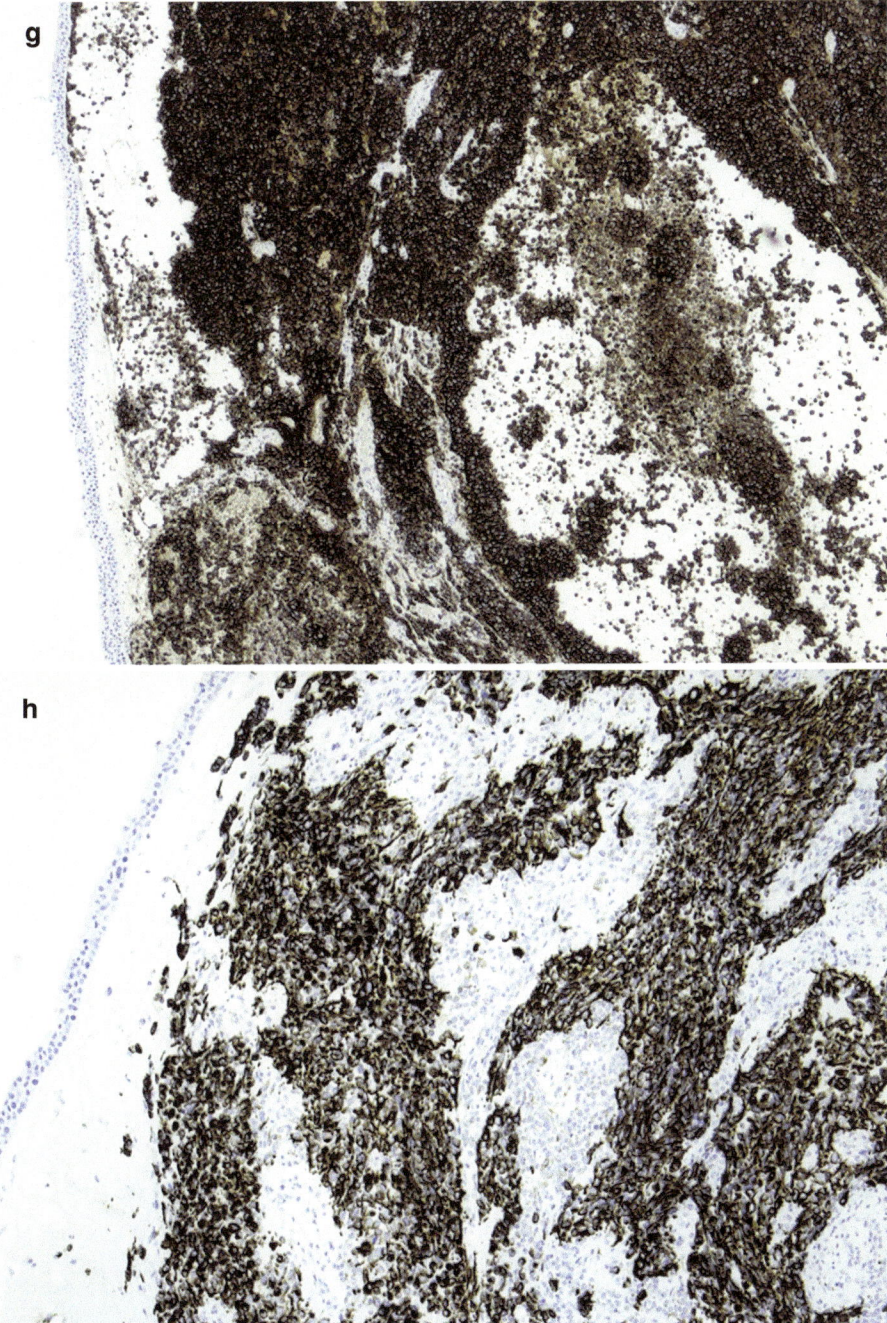

Fig. 3.10 (continued)

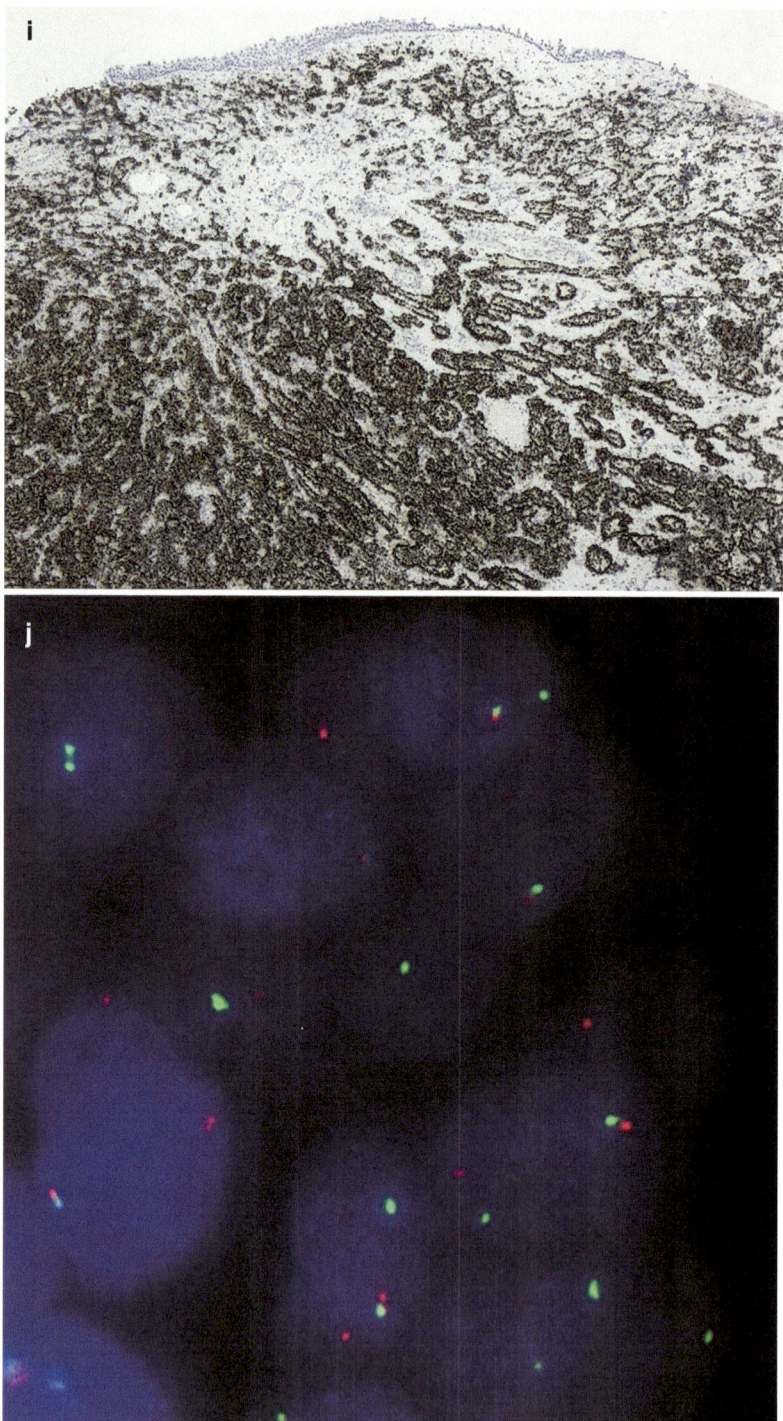

Fig. 3.10 (continued)

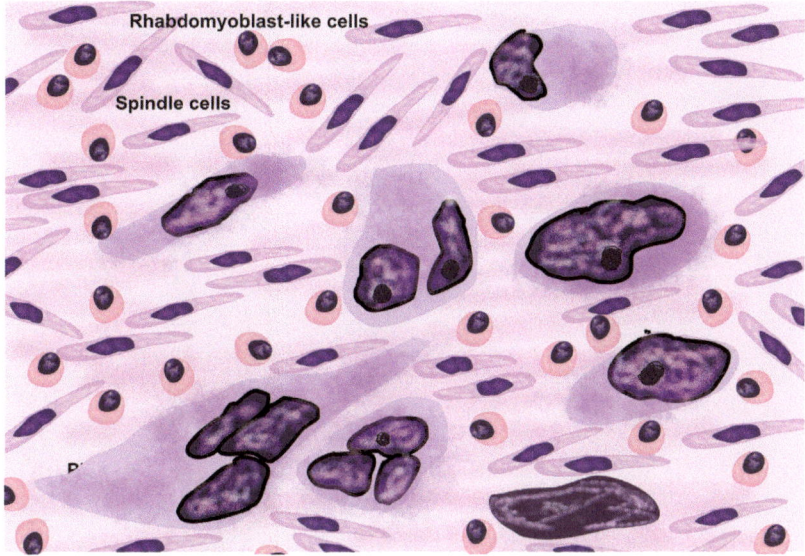

Fig. 3.11 Schematic representation of pleomorphic RMS: spindle cells, rhabdomyoblasts-like cells, and atypical large cells

Pleomorphic Rhabdomyosarcoma (Fig. 3.11)

Definition A rare, high-grade pleomorphic sarcoma of soft tissues, with often minimal skeletal muscle differentiation and typically presenting in older adults.

Age at Presentation >65 years.

Gender Men are more affected than females.

Localization Lower limbs are most frequently involved.

Clinical Course Painful mass, mainly located in the deep soft tissues of the lower limbs.

Macroscopy Well-circumscribed mass, reddish-brown in color, with hemorrhages and necrotic areas on cut surface.

Microscopy Spindled and highly pleomorphic tumor cells dominate the picture, with occasional rhabdomyoblast-like cells. Tumor cells are haphazardly arranged. Pleomorphic cells are characterized by bizarre nuclei, prominent nucleoli, and striking cytoplasmic eosinophilia. Cells with cross striations are rarely encountered (Fig. 3.12a, b).

Immunohistochemistry Nuclear reactivity of atypical tumor cells for myogenin can be very focal (Fig. 3.12c). Desmin is usually more prominent (Fig. 3.12d).

Molecular Genetics Non-diagnostic and non-consisting complex changes.

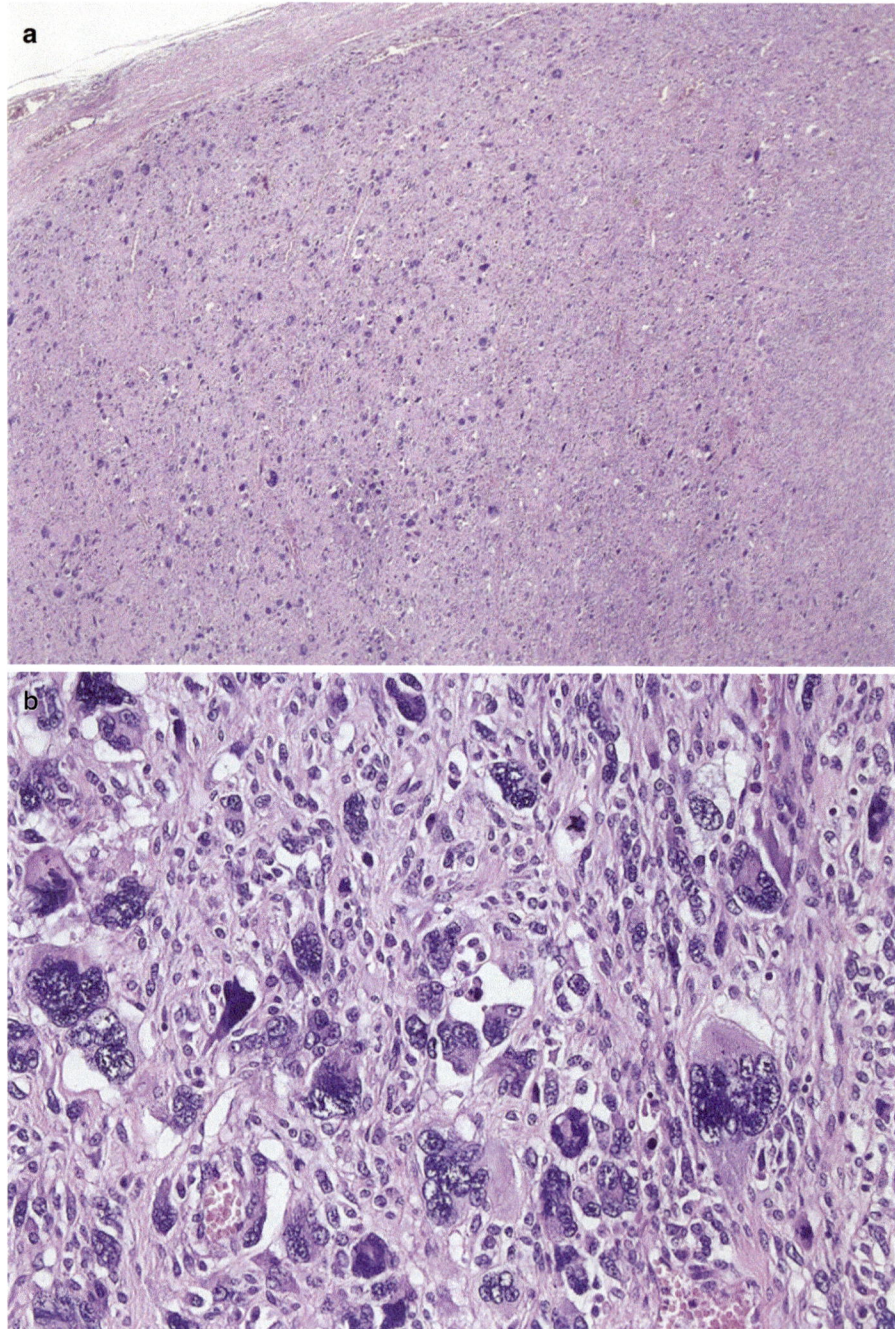

Fig. 3.12 (**a**): Low power field of pleomorphic RMS, from a tumor in the psoas muscle of a 77-year-old male. (**b**): High power field of pleomorphic RMS, characterized by spindle and pleomorphic tumor cells, which show bizarre nuclei and prominent nucleoli. (**c**): Desmin expression pleomorphic RMS. (**d**): Myogenin positivity in pleomorphic RMS

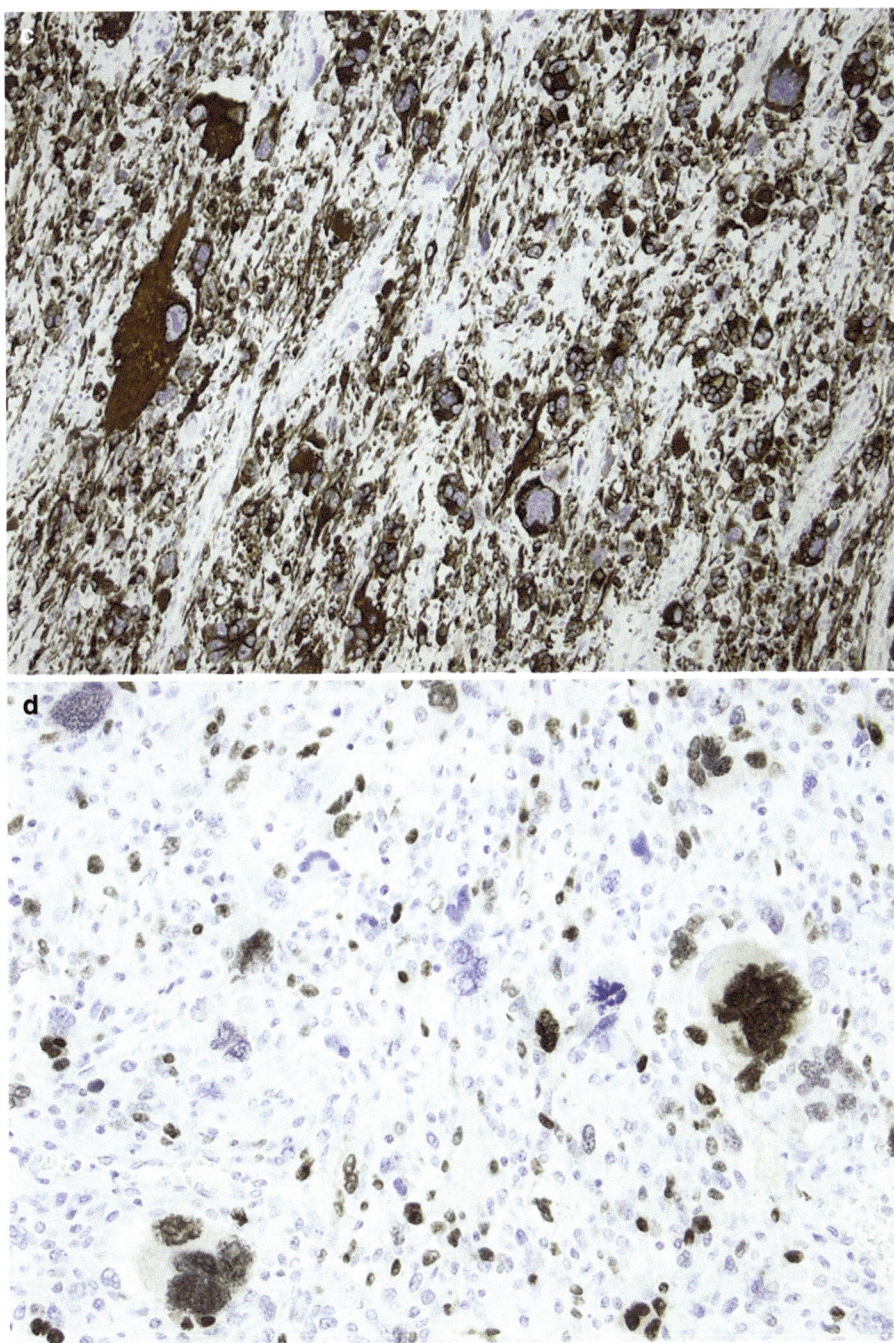

Fig. 3.12 (continued)

Prognosis Pleomorphic RMS is one of the most aggressive pleomorphic sarcomas, with a median survival of 7.3 months.

Differential Diagnosis Any pleomorphic sarcoma and sarcomas with heterologous rhabdomyoblastic differentiation such as *dedifferentiated liposarcoma* and pleomorphic *leiomyosarcoma*. The first shows MDM2 expression/amplification, the second is myogenin negative.

Spindle Cell/Sclerosing Rhabdomyosarcoma (Fig. 3.13)

Definition A rare (5–10%) subtype of RMS, most frequent in early childhood, characterized by a favorable prognosis, and an adult type which is more aggressive.

Age at Presentation Young children (< 10 years) and adolescents. Rare cases in adults.

Gender Male predominate, particularly in childhood.

Localization Paratesticular region> head and neck in children. In adults, head and neck> extremities> trunk.

Clinical Course Superficial/submucosal or deep-seated tumor mass.

Macroscopy Nodular or lobulated mass, fleshy on cut surface.

Microscopy Long intersecting fascicles of eosinophilic spindle cells, often giving rise to a fibrosarcoma- or leiomyosarcoma-like picture. Nuclei are elongated, with vesicular chromatin, indistinct cell borders. Mitotic activity is prominent (Fig. 3.14a–c).

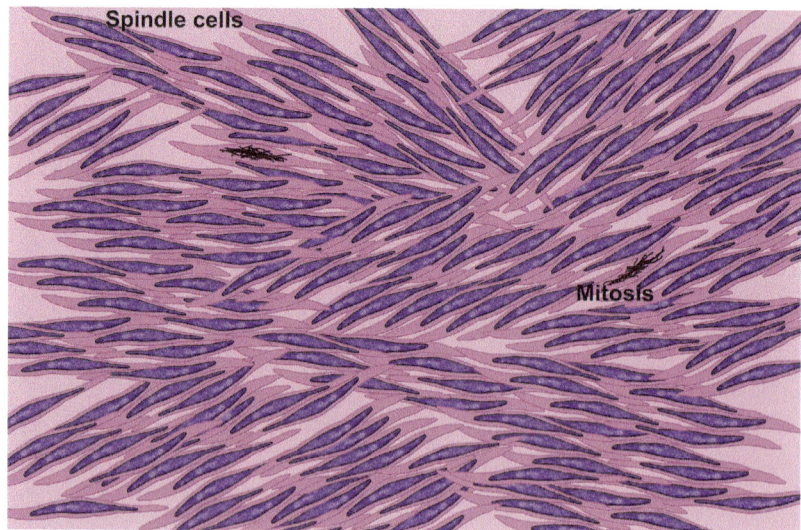

Fig. 3.13 Schematic representation of spindle cells/sclerosing RMS showing the spindle cells and collegenous matrix

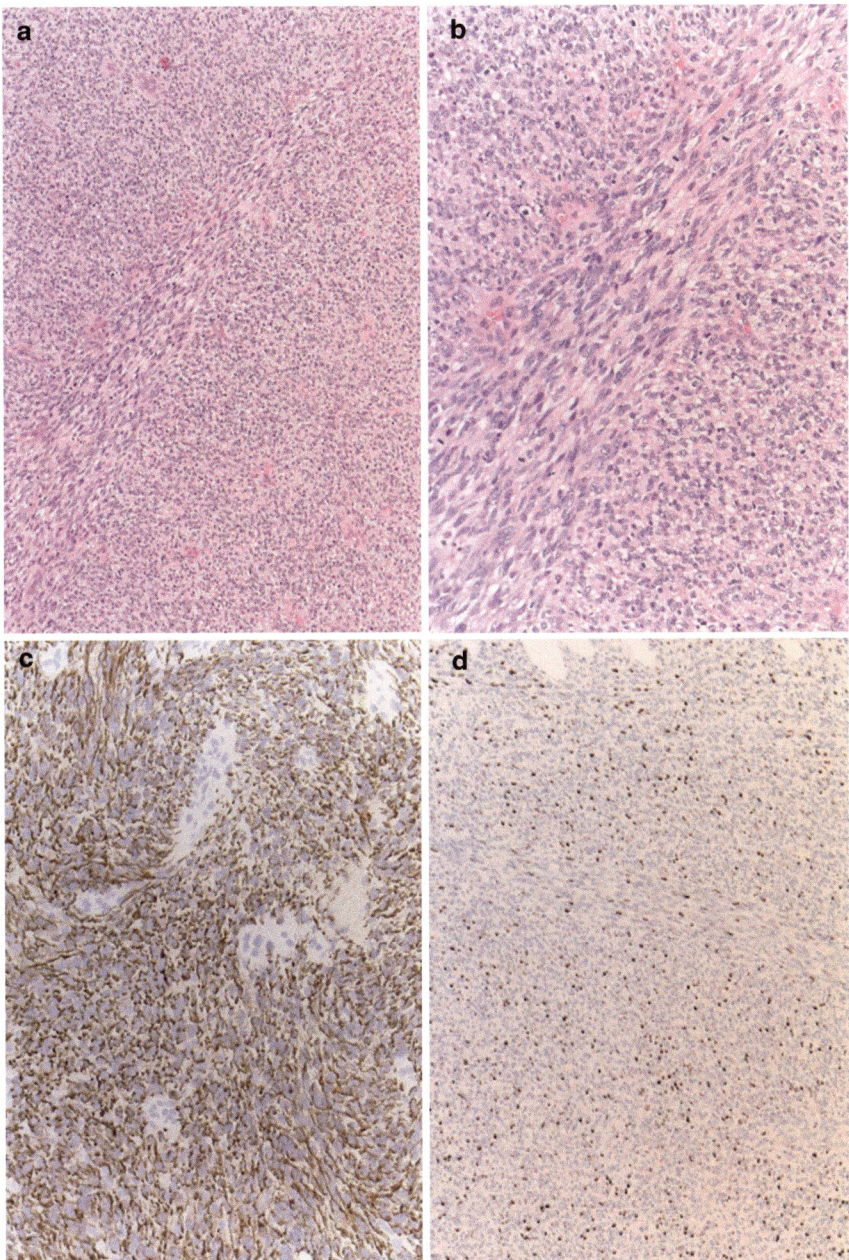

Fig. 3.14 (**a, b**) Spindle cell pediatric RMS from a tumor in the paravertebral muscles and gluteus of a 4-year-old girl, at low power field (**a**) and high power field (**b**) showing compact intersecting fascicles of spindle cells (**c, d**): Immunohistochemistry for desmin (c left side) and myogenin (d right side) in spindle cell pediatric RMS. (**e**): Adult type of spindle cell RMS at low power field, from a tumor in the upper leg of a 56-year-old male. (**f**): Adult type of spindle cell RMS at high power field. Note the rhabdomyoblasts. (**g**): Myogenin expression in adult type of spindle cell RMS

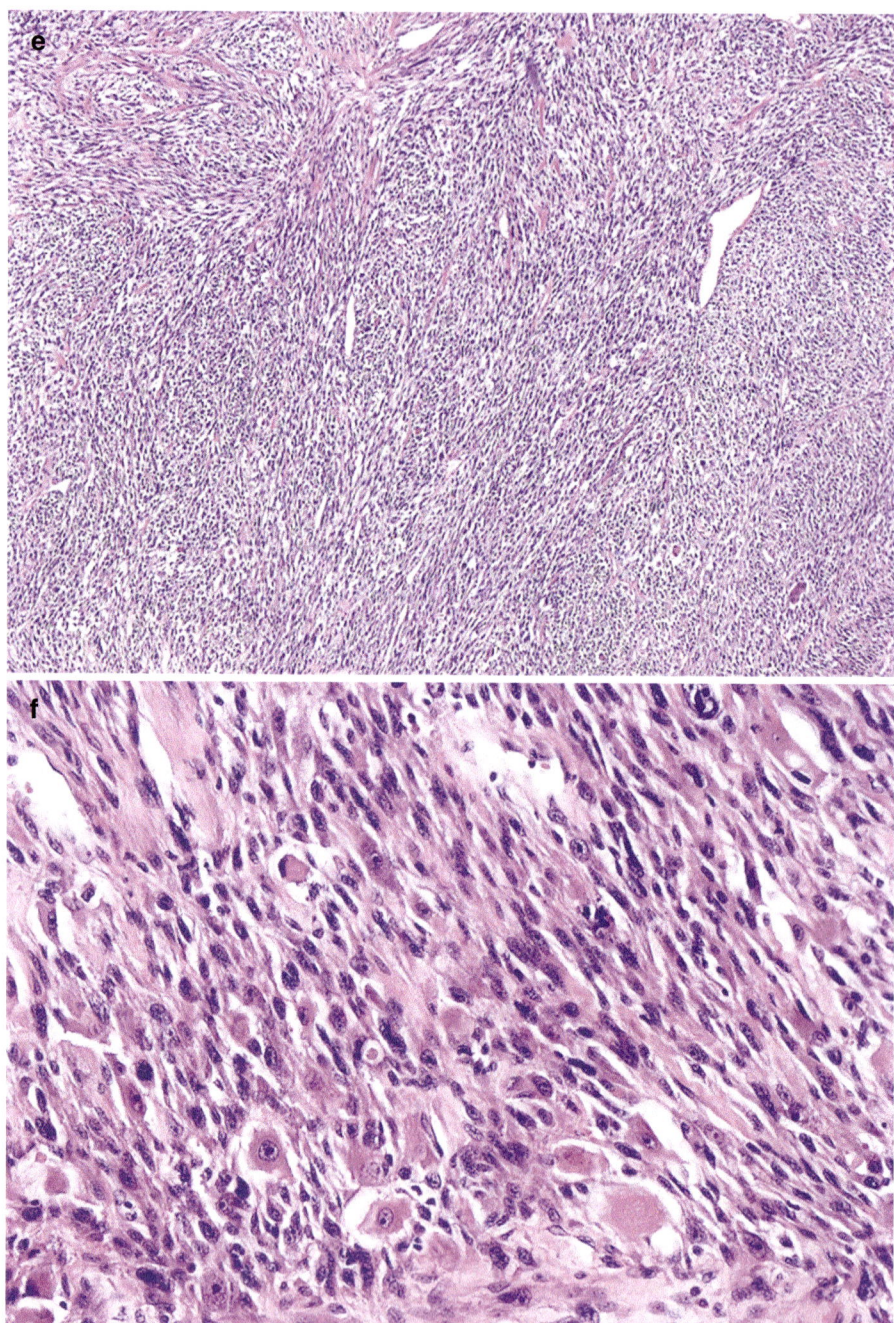

Fig. 3.14 (continued)

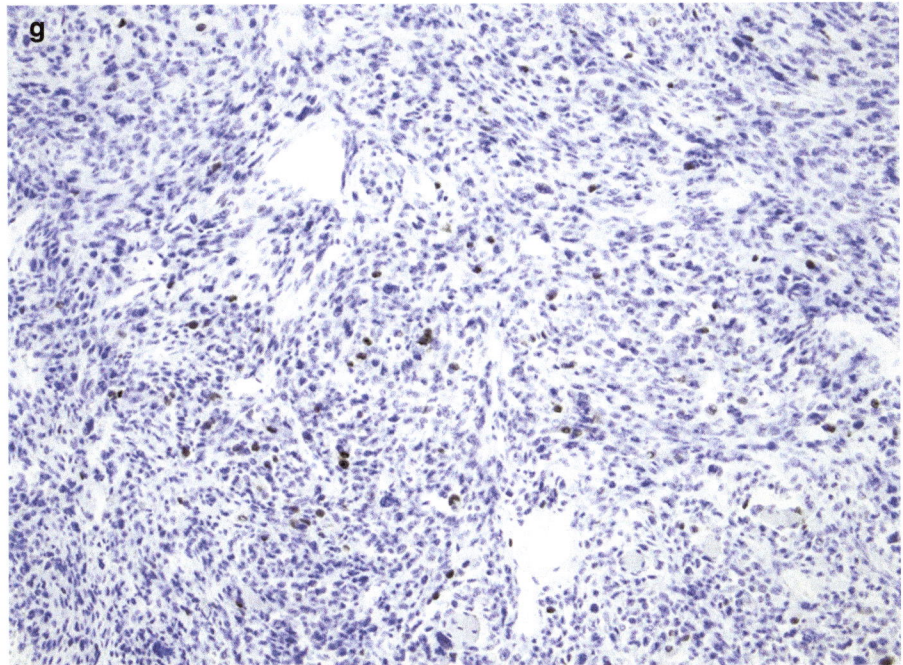

Fig. 3.14 (continued)

Occasional rhabdomyoblasts are seen. The sclerosing variant is characterized by a dense hypocellular, hyalinized eosinophilic stroma, in which spindle tumor cells are arranged in nests or cords and rarely in pseudoalveolar structures.

Immunohistochemistry Spindle cells show immunoreactivity for myogenin and desmin (Fig. 3.14d–g). If MYOD1 mutations are present, expression of this protein is often prominent.

Molecular Genetics There are four genetic subgroups. (1) *NCOA2* and *VGLL2* gene rearrangements in the congenital/infantile spindle cell type. (2) *MYOD1* mutations in the spindle cell/sclerosing type of adolescents/young adults. (3) Spindle cell/sclerosing type without recurrent genetic alterations. (4) Rare intraosseous spindle cell/epithelioid type with *EWSR1/FUS-TFCP2* or *MEIS1-NCOA2* fusion.

Prognosis The overall prognosis of the congenital/infantile spindle cell type with gene fusions is very favorable, with a 5 year survival rate greater than 90%. The MYOD1 mutated type is very aggressive with a 4 year survival rate of 18%.

Differential Diagnosis (1) *Spindle cell (sarcomatoid) squamous cell carcinoma*: reactivity for keratin and p63; (2) *Desmoplastic spindle cell melanoma*: strongly reactive for S100 protein, but negative for HMB45 and Melan-A; (3) *Leiomyosarcoma*: h-caldesmon and smooth muscle actin expression but no myogenin; (4) *Malignant peripheral nerve sheath tumor:* a clinical history of neurofibromatosis type I and loss of H3K27me3 expression; (5) *Synovial sarcoma* (monophasic): expression of TLE1, EMA, and keratin, t(X;18). (6) *Congenital/ infantile fibrosarcoma:* desmin and certainly myogenin expression are no hallmarks; (7) *Sclerosing epithelioid fibrosarcoma: no expression of myogenic markers and presence of MUC-4*

Malignant Ectomesenchymoma (MEM)

Definition It is a rare pediatric mixed sarcoma, composed of a rhabdomyosarcoma, associated with a neuroectodermal tumor, showing differentiation towards neuro- blastoma or ganglioneuroma/ganglioneuroblastoma.

Age at Presentation The highest incidence is in children under the age of 5 years.

Gender No sex predilection.

Localization The pelvis and the paratesticular region are the more frequent site of origin.

Clinical Course A tumor mass, with infiltrative margins, mainly located in the pelvic region.

Macroscopy Single mass localized in the pelvis or paratesticular region.

Histology Fascicles of atypical spindle cells, admixed rhabdoid cells, and with scattered voluminous ganglion cells or neuroblasts.

Immunohistochemistry Tumor cells of the rhabdomyosarcomatous component stain for desmin and myogenin. The neuronal/neuroblastic component is high- lighted by synaptophysin.

Molecular Genetics *HRAS* mutations are frequently found.

Prognosis The overall prognosis is comparable to embryonal rhabdomyosarcoma.

Potential New Entities

In 2019, Martinez et al. described a distinctive rhabdomyoblastic tumor with a prominent histiocytic component and desmin-/myogenin-/MYOD1-positive atypi- cal rhabdomyoblasts. The tumors occurred in adults and were benign. A novel genetic finding was very recently described in three cases with a fusion of the *SRF* gene with *FOXO1* or *NCOA1*. The position of these tumors in the classification of skeletal muscle tumors awaits further study. Among the rhabdomyosarcomas with epithelioid features, there is a predominantly intraosseous variant, with mainly

TFCP2 fusions (see genetics of spindle cell/sclerosing rhabdomyosarcoma). There remains, however, a group of aggressive and prominently epithelioid tumors, mainly occurring in elderly patients. The genetic background of this rare variant is not known.

Tricks for a Correct Diagnosis of Skeletal Muscle Tumors

1. Benign ones are extremely rare.
2. Embryonal rhabdomyosarcoma is the most frequent sarcoma of childhood and the most frequent type of rhabdomyosarcoma.
3. The spindle cell/sclerosing type is a new entity.
4. Rhabdomyoblastic differentiation does not equal rhabdomyosarcoma (MPNST, dedifferentiated liposarcoma, biphenotypic sinonasal sarcoma, nefroblastoma, carcinosarcoma, malignant phyllodes tumor can also contain these cells).
5. Cells with abundant eccentric eosinophilic cytoplasm are not always rhabomyoblasts. Rhabdoid cells can be seen in proliferative fasciitis, myxofibrosarcoma, myoepithelioma, plasmacytoma.
6. Cross striations are very rarely detected in skeletal tumors, so their search is not a practical approach to the diagnosis of skeletal muscle tumors.
7. Myogenin (MYF4) is the most sensitive and specific marker for rhabdomyoblastic differentiation (=nuclear transcription factor involved in striated muscle differentiation).
8. Myogenin expression is retained in degenerated skeletal muscle fibers and should not be mistaken for tumor cells.
9. Alveolar rhabdomyosarcoma is more diffusely positive for myogenin than embryonal rhabdomyosarcoma.
10. Myogenin expression can be very focal in pleomorphic rhabdomyosarcoma.
11. MYOD1 (MYF3) is an alternative transcription factor for striated muscle differentiation and is the most sensitive marker for the MYOD1-mutated variant of adult spindle cell rhabdomyosarcoma.
12. Desmin expression is very sensitive but not specific.
13. Smooth muscle actin can be present, but h-caldesmon is usually not.
14. Alveolar RMS, MYOD1-mutated spindle/sclerosing RMS, and pleomorphic RMS have a poor prognosis.
15. Embryonal RMS and spindle/sclerosing RMS lacking genetic abnormality have a good prognosis.
16. Fusion-positive infantile spindle RMS have a very good prognosis.

Essential References

1. Goldblum JR, Folpe AL, Weiss SW. Enzinger & Weiss's soft tissue tumors. 7th ed. Philadelphia: Elsevier; 2020.
2. Hornick JL. Practical soft tissue pathology: a diagnostic approach: Pattern Recognition Series. 2nd ed. Philadelphia: Elsevier Health Sciences; 2017.

3. Rudzinski ER, Anderson JR, Hawkins DS, Skapek SX, Parham DM, Teot LA. The World Health Organization. Classification of skeletal muscle tumors in pediatric rhabdomyosarcoma. Arch Pathol Lab Med. 2015;139(10):1281–7.

4. Lindberg MR, Chang A. Diagnostic pathology: soft tissue tumors. Philadelphia: Elsevier Health Sciences; 2015.

5. Sunw CB, Wang Y, Stevenson HS, Edelman DC, Meltzer PS, Barr FG. Distinct methylation profiles characterize fusion-positive and fusion-negative rhabdomyosarcoma. Mod Pathol. 2015;28(9):1214–24.

6. Faa G, Sciot R. Soft tissue tumors occurring in the perinatal/infancy setting: 1st part. J Pediatr Neonatal Individ Med. 2018;7(1):e070114.

7. Skapek SX, Ferrari A, Gupta AA, Lupo PJ, Butler E, Shipley J, Barr FG, Hawkins DS. Rhabdomyosarcoma. Nat Rev Dis Prim. 2019;5:1.

8. Agaram NP, LaQuaglia MP, Alaggio R, Zhang L, Fujisawa Y, Ladanyi M, Wexler LH, Antonescu CR. MYOD1-mutant spindle cell and sclerosing rhabdomyosarcoma: an aggressive subtype irrespective of age. A reappraisal for molecular classification and risk stratification. Mod Pathol. 2019;32(1):27–36.

9. Sciot R. Skeletal muscle tumors. In: Folpe AL, Inwards CY, editors. Bone and soft tissue pathology (a volume in the series foundations in diagnostic pathology). 2nd ed: Saunders Elsevier, Philadelphia; 2020, in press.

10. WHO Classification of Tumours Editorial Board. Soft tissue and bone tumors. Lyon: IARC Press; 2020.

Index

© Springer Nature Switzerland AG 2020
R. Sciot et al. (eds.), *Adipocytic, Vascular and Skeletal Muscle Tumors*, Current
Clinical Pathology, https://doi.org/10.1007/978-3-030-37460-0